Department of Health
Welsh Office
Scottish Office Home and Health Department
Department of Health and Social Security, Northern Ireland

Report on Confidential Enquiries into Maternal Deaths in the United Kingdom 1988–1990

Bryan M Hibbard MD PhD FRCOG
Mary M Anderson MB ChB FRCOG
James O Drife BSc MD FRCSEd FRCOG
John R Tighe BSc MD FRCP FRCPath
Sir Keith Sykes MB BCir MA FRCA HonFANZCA
HonFFA(SA)
George Gordon MB ChB FRCSEd FRCOG
John H M Pinkerton CBE DScHonNUI MD FRCOG FRCPI
Dawn Milner MB BS MRCGP
Beverley Botting BSc

London: HMSO

ISBN 0 11 321691 2

CONTENTS

Editorial Board		iv
Preface		vi
Method of Enquiry and Definitions		xi
Glossary of Terms and Abbreviations		xvi
Chapter 1	Trends in maternal mortality	1
Chapter 2	Hypertensive Disorders of Pregnancy	22
Chapter 3	Antepartum and Postpartum Haemorrhage	34
Annexe to Chapter 3 — Revised Guidelines for the Management of Massive Obstetric Haemorrhage		43
Chapter 4	Thrombosis and Thromboembolism	45
Chapter 5	Amniotic Fluid Embolism	55
Chapter 6	Early Pregnancy Deaths	61
Chapter 7	Genital Tract Sepsis Excluding Abortion	73
Chapter 8	Genital Tract Trauma	77
Chapter 9	Deaths Associated with Anaesthesia	80
Annexe to Chapter 9 — Adult Respiratory Distress Syndrome		97
Chapter 10	Other Direct Deaths	100
Chapter 11	Cardiac Disease	106
Chapter 12	Other Indirect causes of maternal deaths	112
Chapter 13	Caesarean section	130
Chapter 14	Fortuitous Deaths	139
Chapter 15	Late Deaths	142
Chapter 16	Pathology	148
Chapter 17	Recommendations	161
Chapter 18	Maternal Mortality in Europe	169
Acknowledgements		178

Editorial Board

| Dr Margaret Hally) | Scottish Office Home and | |
| Dr Sheila Lawson) | Health Department | |

| Dr Adrian Mairs | Department of Health and Social Services | Northern Ireland |

Observers

| Mr J Sharpe) | Department of Health | England |
| Miss J Greenwood OBE) | | |

PREFACE

United Kingdom Confidential Enquiries Into Maternal Deaths
Report 1988-1990

We welcome this second combined United Kingdom (UK) Report of the
Confidential Enquiries Into Maternal Deaths which we believe will be
essential reading for all those involved in the purchasing and provision
of maternity services. In this triennium 325 maternal death report forms
were submitted to the Enquiry. When *Late* and *Fortuitous* deaths are
excluded the reported number of *Direct* and *Indirect* deaths, which con-
form with the International Classification of Diseases definition of
maternal death, was 238 compared with 223 in the previous triennium.
Given the increase in the number of maternities over the period, the
maternal mortality rate has not changed between the two triennia.

The publication of this Report looks at one end of the spectrum of what,
for the great majority of women, is a natural and uncomplicated process.
We believe that the Enquiry serves as a timely reminder of the need for
constant vigilance and expertise in the management of all women so that
the minority who develop serious problems receive appropriate treatment. Above all it is vital that all professionals involved in the provision of maternity services hold paramount the safety of the women and
babies entrusted to their care.

It is disappointing to have to report that this Enquiry has found evidence of substandard care in nearly half of the reported cases of *Direct*
and *Indirect* deaths, a similar finding to that of the previous Report.
Substandard care is defined in the next section of this Report, and it
should be remembered that some circumstances connected with the care
of a woman are outside the control of the clinician. However, the Report
draws attention to the significant number of cases where major problems
were handled by junior doctors, a recurring theme of recent Reports.

We must also draw attention to the levelling since 1985 of the previously downward trend in the maternal mortality rate. Table 1.2 compares the maternal mortality rates per 100,000 maternities derived from
Confidential Enquiry statistics and from figures from Registrars General.
It can be seen that figures from Registrars General show a consistent
maternal mortality rate of seven per 100,000 for the last three triennia
whereas Confidential Enquiry statistics, which include more deaths
than are identified by OPCS coding alone, show a maternal mortality

rate per 100,000 maternities of 11 in the 1982–84 triennium and ten in the two following triennia. This is discussed in more detail in Chapter 1.

Table 1.14 shows that the main causes of *Direct* maternal deaths remain thrombosis and thromboembolism, hypertensive disorders of pregnancy and haemorrhage. The numbers of deaths from hypertensive disorders of pregnancy and from thrombosis and thromboembolism have not altered appreciably between the two triennia. There is evidence that messages relevant to the management of both these causes of maternal death have not been uniformly heeded. A review of certain recommendations made in previous Reports was undertaken by Professor Hibbard and Dr Milner. The findings of this review, which is to be published in Health Trends, and is referred to in Chapters 2 and 3, show that there is still room for improvement in the provision of important facilities. We endorse the recommendation that there should be further research into methods of prevention of thromboembolic complications. We also draw attention to the guidelines on the management of thrombosis which are referred to at the end of Chapter 4.

Sadly, maternal deaths due to haemorrhage have doubled since the previous triennium. It is of particular concern that care was considered substandard in more than half of these cases and that there was, once again, criticism of the level of expertise available for high risk cases. If haemorrhage and ectopic pregnancy deaths are combined they account for 25% of *Direct* maternal deaths (37 out of 145). Looked at in this way, haemorrhage is revealed as the major cause of maternal death. We therefore welcome the revised guidelines on the management of massive obstetric haemorrhage, which are also relevant to the management of ectopic pregnancy, and are included as an annexe to Chapter 3. We are grateful for the advice of Dr A Napier who contributed to this revision.

Sepsis remains a persistent cause of maternal death and both the number and rate of such deaths has nearly doubled since the last triennium. When post abortion sepsis deaths are combined with those of the women who developed sepsis after surgery or after spontaneous delivery, they account for nearly 9% of *Direct* maternal deaths. As is pointed out in Chapter 7, the risk of infection should always be kept in mind.

Chapter 1 presents a statistical overview of data for this triennium and demographic trends relevant to maternal mortality.

Chapters 2 to 13 of the Report consider in detail the 238 *Direct* and *Indirect* deaths for which a completed report form was received. Chapters 14 and 15 discuss *Fortuitous* and *Late* deaths. We endorse the decision to continue collecting data on *Late* maternal deaths which, with improvement in life support techniques, may well be related to an obstetric cause.

Chapter 9 is a thorough and detailed analysis of the circumstances connected with the four "Anaesthetic" deaths and the small group of women where the anaesthetic was thought to have contributed to the death. It is very rewarding to see that the downward trend in deaths due directly to anaesthesia has continued. The rate per million maternities has fallen from 10.5 in the 1973–1975 triennium to 1.7 in this triennium. A useful annexe to this Chapter discusses Adult Respiratory Distress Syndrome (ARDS), which was present in 18.5% of the *Direct* and *Indirect* maternal deaths reported in this triennium.

Chapter 16 reviews available autopsy findings and once again highlights the problem of substandard autopsy reports. We share the view that appropriate further examinations should be undertaken as a matter of routine in all cases of *Direct* and *Indirect* maternal death. We recommend careful consideration and application of the essential requirements for a maternal autopsy which are set out in this chapter.

We encourage readers, in particular all those involved in both the purchasing and provision of maternity services, to pay close attention to the recommendations in Chapter 17. The evidence of this Report is that there are still lessons to be learnt and re-learnt, and for this reason we support the continuation of this important Enquiry.

Chapter 17 also highlights the problems that have been experienced in this triennium in relation to data collection, when, despite repeated requests, information was not provided for 14 known maternal deaths, thereby reducing the coverage of this audit from 99.6% in the last triennium to 96% in this triennium. We wholeheartedly endorse the suggested modification to the death certificate form in England, Wales and Northern Ireland.

This Report includes an incidental chapter entitled Maternal Mortality in Europe (Chapter 18) which is both relevant and timely. We are grateful to Professor Hibbard for collecting the information and writing the chapter, and to all those colleagues in Europe who provided information in response to his questionnaire. It is our hope that this will be a spur to the collection and publication of more accurate data which will permit valid comparisons between the countries of Europe.

Some minor presentational changes are incorporated in this Report. The Foreword has been replaced by an introductory section entitled Method of Enquiry and Definitions, which describes the origin and process of the UK Enquiry and includes definitions previously found in an appendix. It is followed by a glossary of terms and abbreviations which is another new feature.

Appendix A of the 1985–1987 Report contained tables A1, A2 and A3 which listed maternal deaths by OPCS code. The Editorial Board decided to discontinue these three tables, as it was considered that they were no longer of value. The data from the remaining tables A4 to A7 are incorporated into tables presented in Chapter 1, Trends in Maternal Mortality.

We would like to thank the members of the Editorial Board - which at first met under the Chairmanship of Dr Jeremy Metters (Deputy Chief Medical Officer of the Department of Health) and subsequently of Dr Eileen Rubery, Head of the Department's Health Promotion (Medical) Division - and the medical secretary to the Board, Dr Dawn Milner. A list of the members of the Editorial Board is to be found at the beginning of this Report.

The Clinical Sub-group members, also listed at the front of the Report, were ably chaired by Professor Bryan Hibbard, and members of this group were responsible for drafting the individual chapters. The authors met to review these drafts and produce a document which was considered by the whole Editorial Board. The statisticians were co-ordinated by Mrs Beverley Botting of the Health Statistics Division of the Office of Population Censuses and Surveys, who also prepared Chapter 1 with its comprehensive set of tables, produced from data extracted from the maternal death report forms for the four countries.

Professor John Tighe, Professor Sir Keith Sykes and Professor Jack Pinkerton have now retired and we are most grateful for their valuable assistance during the last two triennia. We would also like to thank Professor Richard Beard who was of great assistance during the preparation of this and the previous Report and has now handed over the baton to Professor James Drife, and Dr Robin King, anaesthetic assessor for Northern Ireland, who is retiring.

Our thanks are extended to all those who contributed to the individual case reports in England, Wales, Scotland and Northern Ireland. Without the co-operation of Obstetricians, Anaesthetists, Pathologists, Directors of Public Health, Chief Administrative Medical Officers, General Practitioners, Midwives, Coroners and Procurators Fiscal this valuable work could not be undertaken. Regional Assessors in Obstetrics, Pathology and Anaesthetics have been unstinting in their efforts and have all contributed their expertise and time to the assessment of these case reports. In particular, Regional Obstetric Assessors have co-ordinated the collection of assessments from their colleagues, and met to consider a draft of this Report. In this way we have been presented with a unique Report on an important aspect of maternity care.

It is worth remembering that this Enquiry is the longest running and most prestigious clinical audit in the world, and is considered to be the gold standard on which subsequent confidential enquiries have been based. The maternal mortality rate halved every ten years between 1952 and 1984 and Sir Alexander Turnbull gave a valuable overview of maternal mortality in this century in the 1982–1984 triennial Report. Although the actual number of maternal deaths is now small, the death of a mother is always a tragic event for her family and also for those involved in her care. This Report has demonstrated that elements of substandard care related to service provision, appropriate staffing levels, and clinical standards still exist. For this reason we believe the Enquiry should continue the valuable task of highlighting these deficiences, and that there should be wide attention to, and action on, the recommendations contained within the Report.

CMO England Kenneth Calman

CMO Scotland Robert Kendell

CMO Wales Deirdre Hine

CMO Northern Ireland James McKenna

METHOD OF ENQUIRY AND DEFINITIONS

Method of Enquiry 1988–1990

Historical background

This is the second UK Report and replaces the three separate reports for England and Wales, Scotland and Northern Ireland. The England and Wales reports were published at three-yearly intervals from 1952 - 1984. The reports for Scotland were published at different intervals from 1965 - 1985, the last covering both maternal and perinatal deaths. Future issues in the Scottish series will only include statistical data for maternal deaths. Northern Ireland reports were started in 1956 and were published four-yearly until 1967; because of the small number of maternal deaths the next report covered ten years from 1968–1977, and the last report covered the seven year period 1978–1984. The relatively small number of deaths in Scotland and Northern Ireland led to the decision of the four Chief Medical Officers to change to a combined UK Report after 1984. This decision also ensured maintenance of confidentiality. In order to conserve continuity we have again repeated the arrangement of the last Report by giving separate figures for England and Wales and the United Kingdom. This will be discontinued in the next Report.

England and Wales

The responsibility for initiating an enquiry into a maternal death rests with the Director of Public Health (DPH) in England; or in Wales with the Director of Public Health Medicine/Chief Administrative Medical Officer (CAMO) of the District in which the woman was usually resident. An enquiry form (MCW97) is sent to general practitioners, midwives, health visitors, consultant obstetricians and any other relevant staff who had been concerned with the care of the woman.

When all the information about the death has been collected the DPH forwards the form to the appropriate Regional obstetric assessor in England, or the DPHM/CAMO to the Welsh obstetric assessor. The Regional or Welsh anaesthetic assessors review all cases where there had been involvement of an anaesthetist. Every possible attempt is made to obtain full details of any autopsy which is then reviewed by the Regional or Welsh pathology assessors. The assessors add their comments and opinions regarding the cause or causes of death.

The MCW97 form is then sent to the Chief Medical Officer of the Department of Health or the Chief Medical Officer for Wales. The Central assessors in obstetrics and gynaecology, anaesthetics and pathology then review all available recorded facts about each case and assess the many factors that may have led to death.

Scotland

In Scotland, the system of enquiry is similar. However one panel of assessors deals with all cases. Each obstetric assessor is responsible for a geographical area which includes more than one Health Board; there are two anaesthetic assessors, each of whom comments on anaesthetic aspects of cases from one half of the country; and one pathology assessor. The allocation of cases to diagnostic category is undertaken by the full panel of assessors each year.

On receipt in the Scottish Office Home and Health Department (SOHHD), formerly SHHD, of a certificate of maternal death from the General Registrar's Office (Scotland) an enquiry form (MD1) is sent to the Chief Administrative Medical Officer (CAMO) of the Health Board of residence of the woman concerned. As in England and Wales, the CAMO takes responsibility for organising completion of the MD1 form by all professional staff involved in caring for the woman. When this is achieved he passes the form to the appropriate obstetric assessor who determines whether further data are required before the case is submitted for discussion and classification to the full panel of assessors. In cases where an anaesthetic had been given or an autopsy or pathological investigation undertaken he passes the form to the appropriate anaesthetic or pathology assessor for their comments. He then returns the form to the Enquiry Co-ordinator (a Senior Medical Officer) at SOHHD, who retains it from that time until it has been fully considered, classified and used for preparation of the Report. At all times each form is held under conditions of strict confidentiality and is anonymised before being provided to assessors compiling the Report.

Additional information is obtained from statistics collected and analysed by the Information and Statistics Division of the Scottish Health Service Common Services Agency. This is available from routine hospital discharge data collected by general and maternity hospitals. The coverage by Form SMR2, the maternal discharge summary, is now almost universal at 98% of registered births. General practitioners and hospital and community medical and midwifery staff assist in ensuring that deaths occurring at home are included in the Enquiry.

Northern Ireland

Maternal deaths are reported to the Director of Public Health (DPH) of the appropriate Health and Social Services Board, who initiates completion of the maternal death form (MCW2 Rev.2, 1981) by those involved in the care of the patient. All those providing information understand that this is treated in strict confidence. On completion forms are sent to the Department of Health and Social Services. As in Scotland one panel of assessors deals with all cases. The obstetric assessor reviews each case and where an anaesthetic had been given it is passed to the anaesthetic assessor. The details of autopsies are scrutinised by the pathology assessor. The assessors are asked to consider the report, to give their views on classification and indicate whether care was substandard.

Editorial Board

The Editorial Board consists of a clinical subgroup, a statistical subgroup, departmental representatives of the four countries, together with observers from the Deptartment of Health. The Board is chaired by the head of the Health Promotion (Medical) Division of the Department of Health, and the clinical subgroup is chaired by a central assessor. The clinical subgroup is responsible for the final classification of the cause of death and evidence of substandard care (see definition below). Chapters are drafted by members of the Editorial Board.

Strict confidentiality is observed at all stages of the Enquiry, and the identity of the patient is erased from all forms. After preparation of the Report, and before publication, all the maternal death report forms and related documents are destroyed.

Definitions

Cause of death

A single *main* cause of death has been allotted and subsequently classified according to the International Classification of Diseases, Injuries and Causes of Death — ninth revision (ICD9). This was not necessarily the underlying cause of death. Although deaths are assigned to one main cause and counted in the relevant chapter they may be referred to in other chapters; thus a death assigned to hypertensive disorder of pregnancy, in which haemorrhage and anaesthesia also played a part, may be discussed in all three chapters.

Classification of maternal death

There is an international agreement to subdivide causes of obstetric deaths into *Direct, Indirect* and *Fortuitous*, but only *Direct* and *Indirect* deaths are counted for statistical purposes. ICD9 defines *Direct* obstetric deaths as "those resulting from obstetric complications of the pregnant state (Pregnancy, labour and puerperium), from interventions, omissions, incorrect treatment, or from a chain of events resulting from any of the above". *Indirect* deaths are defined as "those resulting from previous existing disease, or disease that developed during pregnancy and which was not due to direct obstetric causes, but which was aggravated by the physiologic effects of pregnancy". *Fortuitous deaths* are deaths from other causes which happen to occur in pregnancy or the puerperium.

Conceptions and pregnancies

It is now customary for the Office of Population Censuses and Surveys (OPCS) to publish annual estimates of conceptions. This is a count of maternities and legal terminations of pregnancies, to mothers resident in England and Wales, based on the estimated year of conception.

An alternative denominator was used in past Reports for the computation of rates where the numerator included deaths occurring early in pregnancy. These included abortions and ectopic pregnancies. The number of pregnancies was estimated by adding the number of conceptions (see above) to the estimated number of ectopic pregnancies and spontaneous abortions admitted to NHS hospitals. In this Report it has been possible to estimate the number of pregnancies based on limited data from English Hospital Episode Statistics combined with Welsh Hospital Activity Analyses (HAA).

Late deaths

ICD9 defines a maternal death as "the death of a woman while pregnant or within 42 days of termination of pregnancy, from any cause related to or aggravated by the pregnancy or its management, but not from accidental or incidental causes". This is in accord with the definition developed by the International Federation of Gynaecology and Obstetrics (FIGO).

In the Confidential Enquiry, however, some deaths have also been included if they occurred between 43 days and one year after delivery or abortion. These *Late* deaths are considered separately in Chapter 15.

Maternities

In this report deaths are usually related to the number of *maternities*. This is a count of the numbers of mothers *delivered* of live or stillborn infants as distinct from the number of *babies* born, which of course includes twins and other multiple births.

Parity

Parity is defined here as the number of previous registrable live and still births. Official Registration data only record parity from legally registrable births within marriage. Therefore to construct a parity distribution of all maternities it is necessary to estimate the allocation of births outside marriage by parity plus some reallocation of births within marriage (Table 1.10). This has been done in England and Wales by using statistics from the General Household Survey, a sample enquiry conducted each year by the Social Survey Division of OPCS currently covering people in approximately ten thousand private households (one in two thousand of the population). Similar estimates for Scotland and Northern Ireland are not routinely produced.

Substandard Care

The term substandard care has been used in this report to take into account not only failure in clinical care, but also some of the underlying factors which may have produced a low standard of care for the patient. This includes situations produced by the action of the woman herself, or her relatives, which may be outside the control of the clinicians. It also takes into account shortage of resources for staffing facilities, administrative failure in the maternity services and the back-up facilities such as anaesthetic, radiological and pathology services. "Substandard" in the context of the Report means that the care that the patient received, or the care that was made available to her, fell below the standard which the authors considered should have been offered to her in this triennium.

GLOSSARY OF TERMS AND ABBREVIATIONS

AIDS	- Acquired Immune Deficiency Syndrome
APH	- Antepartum haemorrhage
ARDS	- Adult Respiratory Distress Syndrome
ARM	- Artificial rupture of membranes
BEST	- British Eclampsia Survey Team
BP	- Blood pressure
CS	- Caesarean section
CS — PERIMORTEM	- ⎫
CS — PLANNED EMERGENCY	- ⎬ See chapter 13
CS — UNPLANNED EMERGENCY	- ⎭
CEMD	- Confidential Enquiries into Maternal Deaths
CTG	- Cardiotocograph
CT (CAT)	- Computerised Axial Tomography
CVP	- Central venous pressure
D&C	- Dilatation and Curettage
DGH	- District General Hospital
DIC	- Disseminated intravascular coagulation
DVT	- Deep vein thrombosis
DIRECT DEATH	- See text above
ECG	- Electrocardiogram
ECLAMPSIA	- See Chapter 2
FH	- Fetal heart
FORTUITOUS DEATH	- See text above

HDU	- High dependency unit
GP	- General Practitioner
HELLP	- Haemolysis, Elevated Liver Enzymes and Low Platelets[1]
ICD	- International Classification of Diseases
ITU	- Intensive Therapy Unit
IUCD	- Intrauterine Contraceptive Device
IUD	- Intrauterine Death
INDIRECT DEATH	- See text above
LATE DEATH	- See Chapter 15
MATERNITIES	- See Chapter 1
MCW 97	- Maternal Death Report Form
OPCS	- Office of Population Censuses and Surveys
PARITY	- See text above
PE	- Pulmonary embolism
PG	- Prostaglandin
PM	- Postmortem
PPH	- Postpartum haemorrhage
PREGNANCIES	- See text above and Chapter 1
RHA	- Regional Health Authority
SB	- Stillbirth
SHO	- Senior House Officer
SR	- Senior Registrar
SUBSTANDARD CARE	- See text above
UK	- United Kingdom
VE	- Vacuum extraction
WBC	- White blood cells

Reference

1. Weinstein L. *American Journal of Obstetrics and Gynecology*. 1982. **142**: 159–167.

CHAPTER 1

Trends in maternal mortality

This chapter presents statistics to place in context the maternal deaths described elsewhere in this Report. Tables 1.1, 1.2, 1.4, and 1.5 contain data drawn from other official sources.

Trends in maternal mortality

Maternal mortality data are usually presented in one of two ways. The first expresses maternal deaths per million women aged 15–44. This denominator assumes that all women of childbearing age are at risk of becoming pregnant. However, it has the advantage of enabling comparison with other causes of women's deaths. Maternal mortality rates calculated in this way (Table 1.1) have fallen faster than the death rates from all causes for women in the same age group. Between 1973–75 and 1988–90 the UK mortality rate for women aged 15–44 fell by 23 per cent from 808 deaths per million women to 626, whereas over the same period the maternal mortality rate fell by 54 per cent from 9 to 4; in 1988–90 maternal deaths comprised 0.7 per cent of all deaths of women in this age group, compared with 1.1 per cent in 1973–75.

Table 1.1 *Mortality rates per million population aged 15-44 years: All causes and maternal deaths (1973–90), United Kingdom*

	Mortality rates per million females aged 15–44 years		
	All Causes	Maternal deaths	% of deaths in the age group that are due to maternal causes
1973–75	807.9	9.0	1.1
1976–78	763.2	7.5	1.0
1979–81	697.2	6.6	1.0
1982–84	641.7	4.7	0.7
1985–87	622.5	4.2	0.7
1988–90	625.9	4.1	0.7

ICD 8th revision: 1973–77, ICD 630–678
ICD 9th revision: 1978–90, ICD 630–676

Source: 1973 The Registrar General's Statistical Review of England and Wales, Part 1.
1974–90 Mortality statistics, cause. Series DH2 Table 2.
1973–90 The Registrar General's Annual Report, Scotland
1973–90 The Registrar General's Annual Report, Northern Ireland.

The second method of calculating maternal mortality rates is the one which will be used throughout the remainder of this Report. It is based on the premise that only pregnant women are at risk of contributing to the maternal mortality statistics. The true denominator for this approach should be the number of women who had been pregnant during the period of the Enquiry. This would include pregnancies resulting in ectopic pregnancy, spontaneous and legal terminations, stillbirth or live birth. As discussed later in this chapter, since the data for some of these outcomes are unavailable or unreliable, previous Enquiry reports used the number of live and still births for the denominator. A closer approximation, however, is the total number of maternities resulting in a live or still birth.

The number of maternities is used rather than the total number of births since this latter statistic is slightly inflated by multiple births. Although multiple births form only a small proportion of all maternities, their number has risen steadily over the past ten years from over 6,000 maternities in 1980 to over 8,000 in 1990. Part of this is due to the increased number of maternities but the use of ovulation induction drugs and assisted conception techniques is also likely to have played a part. While twin births are quite common at about one per cent of all deliveries, the higher order births are much less so.

The change in denominator since the previous Report does not have a large effect on the resulting statistics. In 1988–90 in the United Kingdom there were 2,360,309 maternities compared with 2,374,827 live and still births. As a result the direct maternal mortality rate for the UK based on the Registrars' General data for 1988–90 would have been 7.2 using total births as the denominator, compared with 7.3 based on maternities.

Figure 1.1 shows the maternal mortality rate for each year between 1973 and 1990 based on statistics from the Registrars General. Table 1.2 presents maternal mortality statistics and maternities in England and Wales for every triennium between 1973–75 and 1982–84, and in the United Kingdom for 1985–87 and 1988–90, based on both those maternal deaths known to the Registrars General and those known to the Enquiry. The maternal mortality rate based on statistics from the Registrars General, expressed per 100,000 maternities, fell by 43 per cent over the period, from 11 in 1973–75 to 7 in 1988–90. Statistics based on maternal deaths known to the Enquiry and the differences between these two sources of data will be discussed more fully in the next section of this chapter.

To place these maternal mortality rates in context, it has been estimated elsewhere[1] that maternal deaths per 100,000 births are 640 in Africa, 420 in Asia, and 270 in Latin America, compared with 30 in all developed countries and less than 10 in Northern and Middle Europe. The current rate of 7 per 100,000 births in the United Kingdom (based on statistics from the Registrars General) is consistent with this. For a further discussion of European maternal mortality data see Chapter 18.

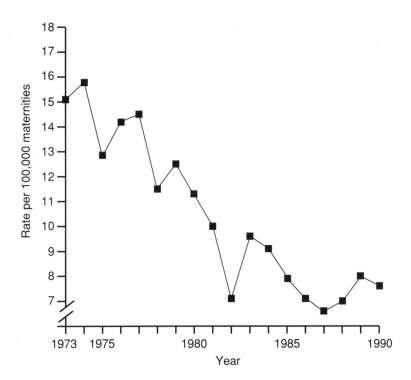

Source: Date from the Registrars General

Maternal deaths known to the Enquiry

In 1988-90 there were 339 deaths known to the Enquiry, but unfortunately, despite repeated requests, completed report forms were not received for 14 of these deaths (compared with one outstanding case in the previous triennium). For the 325 cases in which a completed report form was received, (85 per cent) 277 deaths occurred during pregnancy or before 42 days postpartum (the ICD9 definition of maternal death). The remaining 48 deaths reported for this triennium are classed as *Late* deaths and are considered separately in Chapter 15. The total number of maternal deaths reported to the Enquiry is higher than the number reported in the previous triennium (249 maternal deaths plus 16 *Late* deaths).

A single main cause of death is allocated by the assessors to each maternal death known to the Enquiry. In accordance with the practice established in previous Reports, maternal deaths known to the Enquiry are subclassified into *Direct* deaths resulting from obstetric complications of pregnancy, labour and the puerperium, *Indirect* deaths resulting from either a previous existing disease, or from a disease which developed

3

during pregnancy, and which was aggravated by pregnancy, and *Fortuitous* deaths resulting from causes not related to or influenced by pregnancy. In the current Enquiry there were 145 *Direct* deaths and 93 *Indirect* deaths, a total of 238 maternal deaths where the cause of death was related to the pregnancy and 65 more cases than identified through the Registrars' General statistics.

Table 1.2 *Some statistics of maternal mortality and births 1973–90, England and Wales and United Kingdom*

	England and Wales				United Kingdom	
	1973–75*	1976–78*	1979–81**	1982–84**	1985–87**	1988–90**
Maternities	1,921,568	1,748,851	1,923,725	1,888,753	2,268,766	2,360,309
Maternal deaths known to Registrars General	246	220	201	148	159	173
Maternal mortality rate per 100,000 maternities	13	13	10	8	7	7
Maternal deaths known to Enquiry (Direct and Indirect)	390	325	268	209	223	238
Maternal mortality rate per 100,000 maternities	20	17	14	11	10	10

Figures from Registrars General:
* ICD 8th Revision: ICD 630–678
**ICD 9th Revision: ICD 630–676

Source: England and Wales — 1973–75 Mortality statistics, childhood and maternity, Series DH3, No: 4 table 18.
1976–90 Mortality statistics, cause, Series DH2, table 2.
1964–83 Birth statistics, Series FM1, No.11, table 1.1, 1.2.
1984–90 Birth statistics, Series FM1, No.17, table 1.1, 1.2.
1984–90 Birth statistics, Series FM1, No.17, table 1.1, 1.2.

Table 1.2 showed 173 maternal deaths in 1988–90 recorded from official sources. There are a number of reasons for the different numbers of maternal deaths identified from these two sources. The Registrars' General 173 maternal deaths refer to deaths where the underlying cause of death was "considered to be a complication of pregnancy, childbirth and the puerperium" (ICD9 Chapter XI 630–676). These conditions may have been recorded on other death certificates, but the coding rules led to other conditions on the certificate being given precedence when deriving the underlying cause of death. Also, the woman may have been transferred to a specialist unit when the life-threatening condition arose. Hence, the death may not have been certified by an obstetrician and the original obstetric event not mentioned. To help identify maternal deaths the International Conference on the International Classification of Diseases (10th Revision) suggested that the pregnancy status of women should be collected at death registration. This currently happens in Scotland.

Table 1.3 shows that of the 277 maternal deaths (excluding *Late* deaths) investigated by the Enquiry in 1988–90, 145 (52 per cent) were classified as *Direct*, 93 (34 per cent) as *Indirect*, and 39 (14 per cent) as *Fortuitous*. Data given in the previous Report (56 per cent *Direct*, 34 per cent *Indirect* and 10 per cent *Fortuitous*) showed proportionately more *Direct* deaths and fewer *Fortuitous*.

Table 1.3 also shows that 87 women were known to have died before the twenty-eighth week of their pregnancy; these early maternal deaths comprised a similar proportion (31 per cent) of all maternal deaths as in the previous triennium (30 per cent). Three maternal deaths before 28 weeks gestation resulted in a live birth.

Table 1.3   *Outcome of pregnancy for maternal deaths known to the Enquiry: United Kingdom 1988–90*

	Type of death			
	Direct	*Indirect*	*Fortuitous*	Total
Mole	2	-	-	2
Abortion	10	7	4	21
Under 28 weeks: Ectopic	18	1	-	19
Under 28 weeks: Undelivered	13	14	15	42
Under 28 weeks: Delivered LB	2	1	-	3
Over 28 weeks: Undelivered	7	15	5	27
Over 28 weeks: Delivered	92	54	15	161
Not stated	1	1	-	2
Total	145	93	39	277

NB.   It should be noted that the maternal death may have been subsequent to the end of the pregnancy, and the cause of maternal death may not have been related to the outcome of the pregnancy.

Fertility trends

In order to place these maternal deaths in context, it is important to examine overall fertility trends. Changes in patterns of childbearing could affect the number of maternal deaths. During the 39 years of these Enquiries in England and Wales, and latterly in the United Kingdom, more than 32 million births have been registered in the United Kingdom. Figure 1.2 shows the general fertility rate (births per 1,000 women aged 15–44) over this period, and combined data for each triennium since 1973–75 are given in Table 1.4. The figure shows increasing fertility between 1952 and 1964, peaking in 1964 at 94 births per 1,000 women. This was followed by steadily decreasing rates until 1977 when the general fertility rate reached a minimum of 59. The rate then fluctuated, but since 1982 there has been a small but sustained increase, reaching 64 in 1990. Table 1.4 shows that both the number of births and the birth rate in 1988-90 were higher than those experienced in the previous two triennia.

Table 1.4 *Total number of births (live and still), and fertility rate 1973-90, United Kingdom.*

	Total births (In thousands)	Rate per 1000 women aged 15–44
1973–75	2,239.2	68.8
1976–78	2,038.3	60.9
1979–81	2,235.4	64.2
1982–84	2,183.2	60.7
1985–87	2,293.7	61.9
1988–90	2,374.8	62.5

Source: England & Wales — Birth statistics
      Series FM1 No:11 Table 3.2
         FM1 No:13 Table 1.1, 1.2
         FM1 No:17 Table 1.1, 1.2

      Scotland — Registrar General's Annual Report 1990 Table A 1.3
      Northern Ireland — Registrar General's Annual Report 1990 Table E1.

The small changes in fertility rates since 1977 conceal different influences of a wide range of medical and social changes. Reduced perinatal and infant mortality means that more children are surviving into childhood. There has been an increasing proportion of births outside marriage. This increase has been almost entirely due to an increase in births registered by both parents, which is generally taken to imply that these children are born to parents in a stable relationship. Women on average are older at childbirth, partly due to the greater availability and use of contraceptives, and partly due to older ages at marriage.

Figure 1.2 *General fertility rate, United Kingdom 1952–90*

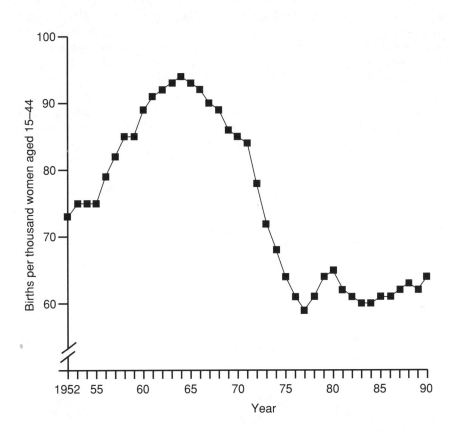

Comparing the component countries of the UK, fertility rates for Northern Ireland are always much higher than other countries but mirror the same pattern. The other three countries have rates close to each other. In Northern Ireland the proportion of births occurring outside marriage is lower than in the other countries. Northern Ireland also has the highest mean age at childbirth. This is due at least in part to women having, on average, more children. In 1990 36 per cent of births within marriage in Northern Ireland were the woman's third or higher order birth, compared with 24 per cent of births in England and Wales.

Trends in legal abortion

Some of the reduction in maternal mortality since 1973 is due to the introduction of legal abortion in 1968 after the 1967 Abortion Act. Since 1970 there has been a consistent decline in deaths from illegal abortion. In 1970–72 (the first full triennium during which legal abortion was available) there were 37 reported deaths from illegal abortion, in 1979–81 there was one, and in the more recent triennia there have been none. The introduction of legal abortion is said initially to reduce and then in the longer term eliminate maternal mortality after illegal abortion[2], and this is supported by these data. The Confidential Enquiry includes deaths of women after spontaneous or legal abortion and investigated three deaths after legal abortion during 1988–90. Between the introduction of the Abortion Act in 1968 in England and Wales and in Scotland, and the end of 1990, over 2 million legal terminations of pregnancy have been carried out on residents of Great Britain. The 1967 Abortion Act does not apply to Northern Ireland where only a small number of legal terminations are performed each year on medical grounds under the case law which applied in England and Wales before the 1967 Abortion Act. However, some women having legal terminations in Great Britain give a usual address in Northern Ireland. This was the case for 5,486 terminations in England and Wales between 1988 and 1990.

Table 1.5   *Legal abortions to women resident in Great Britain, 1970–90*

	No. of Abortions	Rate per 1000 women aged 15–44
1970–72	299,529	9.6
1973–75	351,856	11.1
1976–78	341,191	10.5
1979–81	406,133	12.0
1982–84	420,876	12.0
1985–87	475,330	13.2
1988–90	545,618	15.0

Source: England & Wales — Abortion Statistics, Series AB No 14, table 2

Scotland — Scottish Health Statistics, 1987, –88, –90, table 5.3

Table 1.5 shows both the number of legal terminations in Great Britain and the rate per 1,000 women aged 15–44 for each triennium since 1970–72. The transfer of terminations from the illegal to the legal sector would explain the initial rapid increase in the number of terminations in England and Wales to residents from 22,000 in 1968 to 109,000 in 1972.[3] The number of terminations of pregnancy carried out on residents in Great Britain remained fairly constant until 1978. During the next triennium, 1979–81, there was an increase of almost 65,000 terminations to 406,133, an increase of 19 per cent. Amongst other factors, this increase corresponded with an increase in birth rates. The number of terminations for residents increased in each successive triennium reaching 545,618 in 1988–90. Figure 1.3 shows the legal abortion rate for each individual year over the same period. From 1983 to 1990 there was a continuing upward trend in this rate.

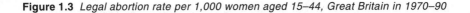

Figure 1.3 *Legal abortion rate per 1,000 women aged 15–44, Great Britain in 1970–90*

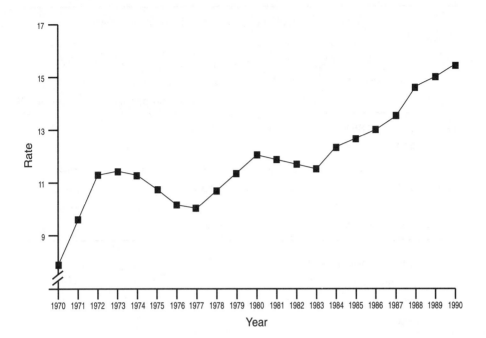

Pregnancies and maternities

As described earlier, due to the unavailability or unreliability of appropriate denominators, in most of the succeeding chapters of this Report maternal deaths will be related to the number of maternities (mothers delivered of live or stillborn infants) rather than to the total number of pregnancies.

In England and Wales the combination of the number of maternities, together with legal terminations, with an adjustment to allow for the period of gestation and maternal ages at conception, provide data which are referred to in official statistics as *conceptions*. The statistics are based on the date of conception. This explains the differences between the data given in Table 1.6 and those given in previous tables in this chapter which are based on the date of delivery. These data are not available routinely for Scotland and Northern Ireland.

Not all pregnancies result in a registrable live or still birth. In Table 1.6 an estimate has been made of the number of *pregnancies*. The number of hospital admissions for spontaneous abortions (at less than 28 weeks gestation) and ectopic pregnancies have been added to the official *conception* statistics. This total is clearly an underestimate of the actual number of pregnancies since these figures do not include other pregnancies which miscarry early, and where the woman is not admitted to hospital, or indeed the woman herself may not even know she is pregnant.

Table 1.6 *Estimated number of pregnancies (in thousands), residents of England and Wales 1973–90*

	Estimated conceptions		Hospital admissions		
	Maternities	Legal abortions	Spont. abortions	Ectopic pregnancies	Total estimated pregnancies
1973–1975	1851.9	327.9	175.3+	11.7	2366.8
1976–1978	1781.3	324.6	158.3+	11.6	2275.8
1979–1981	1910.9	380.5	134.3*	12.1	2437.8
1982–1984	1905.8	393.1	113.6*	14.4	2426.9
1985–1987**	2015.1	451.1	N/A	N/A	2650.9
1988–1990	2073.0	512.7	277.2	24.0	2886.9

+ICD   (8th revision) 640-645

*ICD   (9th revision) 634-638

**Estimated

N/A = Not available

Source: Birth statistics 1837–1983, Series FM1, No: 13, Table 12.2

Birth statistics 1987, series FM1, No: 16

Hospital In-patient Enquiry

England hospital admissions

Wales hospital admissions: Hospital Activity Analysis for Wales

Note: Conceptions statistics are based on date of conception.

The collection of hospital in-patient statistics (HIPE) in England ended after 1985 to be replaced for 1987 onwards by new hospital episode statistics (HES). Unfortunately these data have not been available for all the years covered by this Enquiry. Therefore, an estimate of the number of hospital admissions in England during 1988–90 has been made based on the assumption that the data available are representative of the whole Enquiry period. Welsh data for this triennium were available from the Welsh Hospital Activity Analysis. Using both these sources of data, it is estimated that 72 per cent of pregnancies in England and Wales between 1988 and 1990 led to a maternity resulting in one or more registrable live or still births. A further 18 per cent of pregnancies were legally terminated under the 1967 Abortion Act. The remaining 10 per cent of known pregnancies were admitted to hospital following a spontaneous abortion or an ectopic pregnancy. Spontaneous abortions which resulted in a day-stay or were not admitted to hospital are not included in these data. The changes in the estimated number of spontaneous abortions and ectopic pregnancies between 1982–84 and 1988–90 are likely to be due to the different ways the data were collected during these triennia and the different sampling and grossing up procedures used.

Demographic characteristics of maternal deaths

Regional variation

The wide regional variation in maternal mortality is shown in Table 1.7. The period 1985–90 is used to increase the number of maternal deaths available for analysis. Over the period 1985–90 in the United Kingdom the ratio of *Direct* to *Indirect* deaths was approximately 2:1 but this ratio varied considerably at regional level. In England during this period the direct obstetric maternal mortality rate per 100,000 total births varied between 9.7 per 100,000 births in North West Thames RHA and 3.8 per 100,000 births in Oxford RHA.

Table 1.7 *Direct and Indirect maternal deaths in the Enquiry and mortality rate by area of residence, 1985–90*

Area of residence	Reported			Direct obstetric mortality rate**	Perinatal mortality rate+
	Total births	*Direct deaths**	*Indirect deaths*		
United Kingdom	4,666,120	284	177	6.1	8.9
England	3,876,169	240	143	6.2	8.9
Wales	228,495	17	11	7.4	9.0
Scotland	396,509	23	14	5.8	9.2
Northern Ireland	164,947	4	9	2.4	9.4
Regional Health Authorities					
Northern	242,628	15	7	6.2	9.1
Yorkshire	298,014	17	14	5.7	9.3
Trent	367,790	25	15	6.8	9.2
East Anglia	154,703	10	9	6.5	7.4
North West Thames	297,747	29	4	9.7	8.3
North East Thames	332,592	14	10	4.2	9.1
South East Thames	300,520	21	13	7.0	8.7
South West Thames	230,512	12	8	5.2	7.8
Wessex	223,297	10	2	4.5	8.5
Oxford	209,783	8	10	3.8	7.9
South Western	239,420	14	11	5.8	7.9
West Midlands	436,856	31	21	7.1	10.4
Mersey	199,599	13	10	6.5	8.6
North Western	342,708	21	9	6.1	9.6

* includes abortion
**Per 100,000 total births
+ Stillbirths & deaths under 1 week combined per 1,000 live and stillbirths

Table 1.7 also shows the perinatal mortality rates for each country and for each RHA in England over the same period. These rates, together with the maternal mortality rates, are shown in Figure 1.4 ordered by increasing maternal mortality rates. Whilst West Midlands RHA

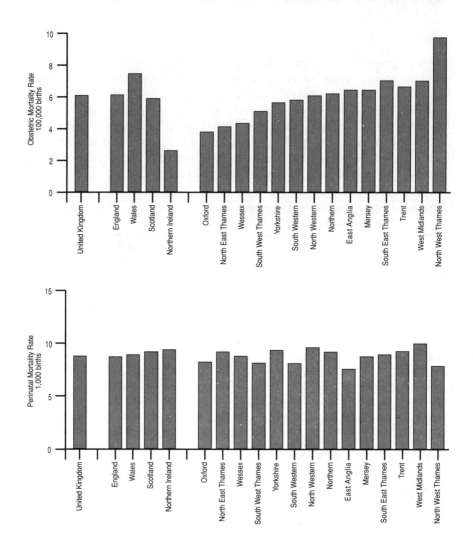

Figure 1.4 *Direct obstetric mortality and perinatal mortality rates, United Kingdom 1985–90*

ranked among the highest rates for both direct obstetric mortality and perinatal mortality, and Oxford RHA ranked among the lowest rates for both categories, other regions showed no consistent pattern. Kendall's rank correlation test showed no statistically significant association (at 5 per cent level) between the ranked order of the direct obstetric mortality rate and that of the perinatal mortality rate.

Age and parity

Maternal mortality is closely related to both maternal age and parity, as shown by the data presented in Tables 1.8 and 1.9. Tables 1.8 and 1.9 replace the table in the previous Report showing maternal deaths cross tabulated by age and parity, and tables given in the appendix of the previous Report. The numbers in each cell of the cross tabulation by age and parity were too small for meaningful analysis. Maternal death rates generally rose with age as shown in Table 1.8. All-cause mortality rates

Table 1.8 *Number of deaths by age of mother in the Enquiry, United Kingdom 1985-90 and the rate per million maternities*

Age	Number of Maternal Deaths 1985–87			Number of Maternal Deaths 1988–90			Rate Per Million Maternities 1985–87			Rate per million maternities 1988–90			Percentage of all deaths to women (in age group) due to maternal conditions
	Direct	Indirect	Fortuitous	Direct	Indirect	Fortuitous	Direct	Indirect	Fortuitous	Direct	Indirect	Fortuitous	
Under 16													
16–17	1		1	4	1	1	62.6*	15.7	5.2	46.6*	41.4*	15.5*	0.2
18–19	11	3	1	5	7	2							1.0
20–24	24	23	5	21	17	4	37.1	35.6	7.7	33.2	26.9	6.3	1.0
25–29	34	19	8	39	35	11	43.7	24.4	10.3	46.6	41.8	13.2	1.8
30–34	36	24	4	39	18	14	82.3	54.9	9.1	78.0	36.0	28.0	1.8
35–39	28	7	3	19	12	3	184.1	46.0	19.7	113.4	71.6	17.9	0.7
40–44	5	6	5	14	2	2	187.7**	225.3**	187.7**	508.4**	63.6**	95.3**	0.2
45+		2		2	0	1							
Not stated				2	1	1							
Total	139	84	26	145	93	39	62.3	37.6	11.6	61.4	39.4	16.5	0.8

* Rates for age under 20
** Rates for age 40 & and over.

13

Table 1.9 *Number of deaths by parity of mother in the Enquiry, United Kingdom 1985-90 and the rate per million maternities*

Parity	Number of maternal deaths 1985–87			Number of maternal deaths 1988–90			Rate per million maternities 1985–87			Rate per million maternities 1988–90		
	Direct	*Indirect*	*Fortuitous*	*Direct*	*Indirect*	*Fortuitous*	*Direct*	*Indirect*	*Fortuitous*	*Direct*	*Indirect*	*Fortuitous*
0	57	30	9	35	22	8	60.9	32.0	9.6	32.5	20.4	7.4
1	28	22	8	30	14	7	37.8	29.7	10.8	41.5	19.4	9.7
2	19	11	2	4	6	7	55.5	32.2	5.8	11.9	17.9	20.8
3	17	10	3	3	2	2	133.1	78.3	23.5	22.8	15.2	15.2
4+	15	11	4	7	6	2	177.4	118.3	47.3	76.5	65.5	21.8
NS	3	–	–	66	43	39	–	–	–	–	–	–
Total	139	84	26	145	93	65	62.3	37.6	11.6	61.4	39.4	16.5

NS = Not stated

14

for women also rose throughout the age group 16–45 but the contribution of maternal causes peaked for ages 25–34, being lowest for women aged under 20 or 40 and over. There was a different pattern of maternal mortality with parity (Table 1.9), with lowest rates for *Direct* deaths being for women in their third pregnancy (parity 2).

Table 1.10 *Percentage distribution of all live births by parity and age, and age at first birth, from 1973–1990, England and Wales only*

	1973–75	1976–78	1979–81	1982–84	1985–87	1988–90
Parity						
0	40	41	41	40	41	41
1	36	37	35	35	34	34
2	14	14	15	16	16	16
3	5	5	5	6	6	6
4 and over	4	3	3	3	3	3
Total	100	100	100	100	100	100
Age (years)						
Under 20	11	10	9	9	9	8
20-24	32	31	31	30	29	27
25-29	37	37	34	34	35	35
30-34	14	17	20	19	20	21
35-39	5	5	5	7	7	7
40 and over	1	1	1	1	1	1
Total	100	100	100	100	100	100
Age (years) at first birth						
Under 20	21	19	18	18	17	16
20-24	39	38	39	38	36	33
25-29	31	32	30	31	32	33
30-34	7	9	11	11	12	14
35 and over	2	2	2	3	3	4
Total	100	100	100	100	100	100

Source: Unpublished OPCS fertility tables.
*Note: Exact parity figures are only available for births inside marriage.
The data in this table are based on estimates of "true" parity order estimated by using information from the General Household Survey.

The pattern of fertility in terms of age and parity has changed over recent years. These changes can make an important contribution to maternal mortality because, as previously discussed, maternal mortality risks become higher with increasing age and parity.

Between 1980 and 1990 fertility rates increased considerably among women in their thirties and forties. In contrast, rates fell among women in their twenties. However, the late twenties remain the peak childbearing years with fertility rates substantially above those for all other age groups.

Table 1.10 shows separately the changes in the age and parity distribution of live births in England and Wales for every triennium between 1973–75 and 1988–90. More women are delaying childbearing. In 1973–75, 60 per cent of women having their first child were aged under 25, whereas by 1988-90 only 49 per cent were aged under 25.

Marital status

One of the most striking trends in recent years has been the dramatic increase in both number and proportion of all births occuring outside marriage, which had risen to 28 per cent of births in the United Kingdom by 1990. The levels in England, Wales and Scotland were very similar (28 per cent, 29 per cent and 27 per cent respectively). However, the proportion of births outside marriage in Northern Ireland (19 per cent), was less than in Great Britain, although the rate of increase over the previous decade was similar[4]. Nevertheless, this increase has been concentrated in births outside marriage registered by both parents, usually giving the same address. During the period 1980 to 1990 the proportion of all births which occurred outside marriage and were registered by the mother alone remained at 6-8 per cent.

Table 1.11   *Maternal deaths in relation to marital status, United Kingdom 1988–90*

Marital status	*Direct* deaths	*Indirect* deaths	Total		Percentage of series
Married	99	60	159		66.8
Single	29	26	55		
Widowed	1	1	2		
Divorced	4	1	5	}	26.9
Separated	2	0	2		
Not stated	10	5	15		6.3
Total	145	93	238		100.0

Table 1.11 shows the marital status of the women who suffered a *Direct* or *Indirect* maternal death in 1988–90. Sixty seven per cent of the women were known to be married at the time of death, which is consistent with the 72 per cent of live births born inside marriage in 1990 in the United Kingdom. This suggests that being unmarried is not in itself a risk factor for maternal mortality overall. Therefore, marital status will not be considered in the later chapters of this Report.

Cause of maternal mortality

Table 1.12 shows the causes of *Direct* maternal deaths and the percentage they formed of all maternal deaths in England and Wales from 1973

Table 1.12 *Causes of Direct maternal deaths, England and Wales 1973–90 and United Kingdom, 1985–90*

		Pulmonary embolism	Hypertensive disease	Anaesthesia	Amniotic fluid embolism	Abortion	Ectopic pregnancy	Haemorrhage	Sepsis, excluding abortion	Ruptured uterus	Other Direct causes	All deaths
England and Wales												
1973–75	No.	33	34	27	14	27	19	21	19	11	22	227
	%	14.5	15.0	11.9	6.2	11.9	8.4	9.3	8.4	4.8	9.7	100
1976–78	No.	43	29	27	11	14	21	24	15	14	19	217
	%	19.8	13.4	12.4	5.1	6.5	9.7	11.1	6.9	6.5	8.8	100
1979–81†	No.	23	36	22	18	14	20	14	8	4	19	178
	%	12.9	20.2	12.4	10.1	7.9	11.2	7.9	4.5	2.2	10.7	100
1982–84	No.	25	25	18	14	11	10	9	2	3	21	138
	%	18.1	18.1	13.0	10.1	8.0	7.2	6.5	1.4	2.2	15.2	100
1985–87	No.	24*	25	5	9	6	11	10	6	5**	20***	121
	%	19.8	20.7	4.1	7.4	5.0	9.1	8.3	5.0	4.1	16.5	100
1988–90	No.	23	25	3	10	7	15	21	6	2	24	136
	%	16.9	18.4	2.2	7.4	5.1	11.0	15.4	4.4	1.5	17.6	100
United Kingdom												
1985–87	No.	29*	27	6	9	6	16	10	6	6**	24§	139
	%	20.9	19.4	4.3	6.5	4.3	11.5	7.2	4.3	4.3	17.3	100
1988–90	No	24	27	4	11	9	15	22	7	2	24	145
	%	16.6	18.6	2.8	7.6	6.2	10.3	15.2	4.8	1.4	16.6	100

* excluding deaths following abortion
** including other genital tract trauma
*** includes 2 thrombosis deaths
† includes 2 other *Direct* deaths omitted in the 1976–78 Report
§ includes 3 deaths from thrombosis and 1 *Direct* cardiac death

to 1990 and in the United Kingdom from 1985 to 1990. Figure 1.5 shows the causes of Direct maternal deaths and their percentages for this triennium. The main causes of death remain the same as in the previous triennium: hypertensive disease, pulmonary embolism, haemorrhage and ectopic pregnancy, which together comprised over 60 per cent of all *Direct* maternal deaths.

Figure 1.5 *Cause of Direct maternal deaths, United Kingdom 1988–90*

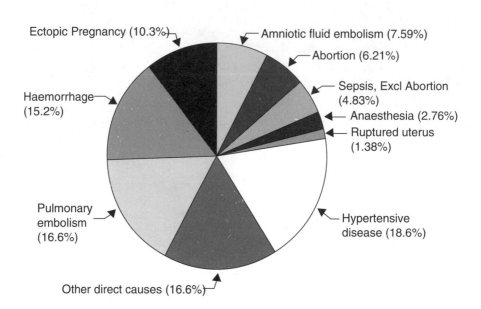

Table 1.13 gives *Direct* maternal death rates per million pregnancies, by cause, for England and Wales from 1973 to 1990.

Table 1.14 is comparable to table 1.12 in the previous Report and shows the new groupings of *Direct* maternal deaths for the UK for the last two triennia. This table demonstrates that thrombosis and thromboembolism remain the major direct cause of maternal death.

Each of the causes of maternal death will be considered separately in the following chapters.

Table 1.13 *Direct deaths by cause, rates per million estimated pregnancies, England and Wales 1973–90†*

Cause of *Direct* maternal death											
	Pulmonary embolism	Hypertensive disorders of pregnancy	Anaesthesia	Amniotic fluid embolism	Abortion	Ectopic pregnancy	Haemorrhage	Sepsis, excluding abortion	Ruptured uterus	Other direct causes	All deaths
1973–75	12.8	13.2	10.5	5.4	10.5	7.4	8.1	7.4	4.3	8.5	88.0
1976–78	18.5	12.5	11.6	4.7	6.0	9.0	10.3	6.5	6.0	8.2	93.4
1979–81*	9.0	14.2	8.7	7.1	5.5	7.9	5.5	3.1	1.6	7.5	70.0*
1982–84	10.0	10.0	7.2	5.6	4.4	4.0	3.6	1.0	1.2	8.4	55.0
1985–87	9.1	9.4	1.9	3.4	2.3	4.1	3.8	2.3	1.9	7.5	45.6
1988–90	8.0	8.6	1.0	3.5	2.4	5.2	7.3	2.1	0.7	8.3	47.0

* Includes two other *Direct* deaths omitted in the 1976-78 Report.

† Rates for the United Kingdom were not available as there was no information on pregnancies for Scotland and Northern Ireland.

Table 1.14 Causes of Direct maternal deaths, United Kingdom, 1985–1987 and 1988–90

Cause of Direct maternal death									
Thrombosis and thrombo-embolism	Hypertensive disorders of pregnancy	Anaesthesia	Amniotic fluid embolism	Early pregnancy deaths (including abortion)	Antepartum and postpartum haemorrhage	Genital tract sepsis (excluding abortion)	Genital tract trauma	Other direct deaths	All deaths
1985–87									
No.									
32*	27	6	9	22	10	6	6	21**	139
%									
23.0	19.4	4.3	6.5	15.8	7.2	4.3	4.3	15.1	100
1988–90									
No.									
33	27	4	11	24	22	7	3	14	145
%									
22.7	18.6	2.8	7.6	16.6	15.2	4.8	2.1	9.7	100

* Excluding 1 death following abortion, but including 3 deaths from thrombosis.

** Including 1 *Direct* cardiac death

References

1. Editorial. Maternal health in Subsaharan Africa. *Lancet* 1987; **i:** 255–257.
2. Högberg U. Maternal mortality — a worldwide problem. *Int J Gynaecol Obstet*, 1985, **23:** 463–470.
3. Botting B. Trends in abortion. *Population Trends*, no **64:** HMSO, (1991).
4. Craig J. Fertility trends within the United Kingdom. *Population Trends*, no **67:** HMSO, 1992.

CHAPTER 2

Hypertensive Disorders of Pregnancy

Summary

There were 27 deaths due to hypertensive disorders of pregnancy in the United Kingdom (UK) during the triennium 1987 to 1990 the same number as in the previous triennium. In only one case was there pre-existing known hypertension; there were 14 cases of eclampsia. The related perinatal mortality fell sharply from a figure of 370 per thousand in the last report to 131.

Substandard care was evident in 88% of cases compared with 81% in the previous Report. Underlying factors were delay in taking clinical action, inadequate control of blood pressure and failure to appreciate, often at too junior a level of clinical responsibility, the seriousness of symptoms and signs.

In only eight cases was the help of a Regional centre sought. Otherwise care at local level had apparently been considered adequate or to have been suddenly overtaken by unforeseen deterioration. In many cases postpartum care was clearly substandard.

Hypertensive disorders of pregnancy are now the main direct cause of maternal death in the UK and the lack of improvement is both disappointing and perplexing. The deaths all occurred before the recommendations of the previous Report were published. The British Eclampsia Survey Team's report (BEST) may give a clearer picture of how eclampsia in particular is being managed at present throughout the United Kingdom.

The clinical classification devised by the International Society for the Study of Hypertension in Pregnancy has been used, but the well established terms "pre-eclampsia" and "eclampsia", which relate to a pregnancy specific syndrome characterised by a group of symptoms of which hypertension is one, have been retained.

The number of women who died from hypertensive disorders of pregnancy and the death rate per million maternities for the years 1973 to 1990 inclusive in England and Wales are compared with those for the United Kingdom from 1985 to 1990 in Table 2.1

Table 2.1 *Number of women who died from hypertensive disorders of pregnancy and the death rate per million maternities, England and Wales 1973–1990, compared with United Kingdom. 1985–1990*

	Total		Pre-eclampsia		Eclampsia	
	Number	Rate	Number	Rate	Number	Rate
England & Wales						
1973–75	34	17.7	15	7.8	19	9.9
1976–78	29	16.6	16	9.1	13	7.4
1979–81	36	18.7	16	8.3	20	10.4
1982–84	25	13.3	11	5.8	14	7.4
1985–87	25	12.6	13	6.5	12	6.0
1988–90	24	11.5	10	4.8	14	6.7
United Kingdom						
1985–87	27	12.1	15	6.7	12	5.4
1988–90	27	11.0	12	5.1	14	5.9

A comparison of the ages of the women who died of a hypertensive disorder of pregnancy in the United Kingdom in 1985–1987 and 1988–1990 is given in Table 2.2. The influence of age is again apparent.

Table 2.2 *Number of maternal deaths and the death rates per million maternities from hypertensive disorders by age, United Kingdom, 1985–1987 and 1988–1990*

Age (years)	1985–87			1988–1990		
	Maternities total (000s)	No of deaths	Rate per million	Maternities total (000s)	No of deaths	Rate per million
Under 25	837.8	10	11.9	825.0	8	9.6
25-29	777.7	5	6.4	836.4	5	5.6
30-34	437.6	7	16.0	499.9	8	16.0
35-39	152.1	3	19.7	169.5	4	23.8
40+	26.6	2	75.1	31.5	2	63.5
All ages	2,231.8	27	12.1	2360.3	27	11.4

Established pre-eclampsia and eclampsia were the sole causes of death in all the 27 cases. In every case but one, the blood pressure was normal in early pregnancy.

In eight other women, severe pre-eclampsia was a significant factor but the deaths were considered to be due to other causes and are therefore counted in the appropriate chapters. The causes were pulmonary thromboembolism, cerebral thrombosis, anaesthesia, post-operative haemorrhage, two of cardiac disease and two of subarachnoid haemorrhage. In this triennium only one woman died undelivered. Her case is described later. There were three *Late* deaths notified to this Enquiry which are counted in Chapter 15.

Duration of Pregnancy

The duration of pregnancy at delivery is shown in Table 2.3.

Table 2.3 *Duration of pregnancy at delivery*

Duration of Pregnancy* (weeks)	Pre-eclampsia	Eclampsia	Total
Up to 28	2	1	3
29–32	2	2	4
33–37	5	7	12
38+	3	4	7
Totals	12	14	26

*One woman died undelivered

Twenty six of the 27 women died after delivery.

Seven of the 27 deaths occurred before 33 weeks gestation, four due to pre-eclampsia and three to eclampsia.

Mode of Delivery

In one case, severe pre-eclampsia developed at 22 weeks, the fetus died and the pregnancy was terminated. One woman died undelivered. Twenty-five pregnancies resulted in 30 births as there were three sets of twins and one triplet pregnancy. There were eight spontaneous vaginal deliveries, including two sets of twins, four infants were delivered by forceps, and 15 by Caesarean section, one with twins and one with triplets.

Perinatal Mortality

Excluding the fetus of the mother who died undelivered there were four intra-uterine deaths. The perinatal mortality, four of 30 total births or a rate of 133 per 1,000 compares with 370 per 1,000 in the previous report. It is notable that all three babies born alive before 28 weeks survived.

Time of first fit

Eclampsia occurred in 14 cases and severe pre-eclampsia in 13. Ten women had their first fit before any specific treatment for pre-eclampsia had been initiated, three of them at home. In none of the women who had their first fit at home had expert medical or paramedical help been obtained. Eleven of the 14 eclamptics suffered fits after admission to hospital and eight of them had more than one fit. This suggests that initial treatment was inadequate and that convulsions were not satisfactorily controlled thereafter.

Table 2.4 *Number and timing of eclamptic fits*

Number of fits	Antepartum	Postpartum	Total women
1	5	2	7*
2	3	3	6
3	1	0	1
8	0	1	1

*One woman had one fit before and one after delivery.

Table 2.4 shows the number and timing of fits. One patient convulsed both before and after delivery.

Immediate Cause of Death

The immediate causes of death in all 27 cases are shown in Table 2.5. There was associated disseminated intravascular coagulation (DIC) in 15 cases.

Table 2.5 *Causes of death UK 1985–90*

Causes of death	1985–87	1988–90
Cerebral	11	14
Haemorrhage-Intracerebral		10
Subarachnoid	11	2
Infarction	0	1
Oedema	0	1
Pulmonary	12	10
Adult Respiratory Distress Syndrome	9	9
Oedema	1	1
Haemorrhage	1	0
Bronchopneumonia	1	0
Hepatic	1	1
Necrosis	1	1
Other	3	2
Total	27	27

In the previous triennium the ratio of deaths from pulmonary complications to deaths from intra-cerebral damage was aproximately 1 to 1. In the present Report the ratio has changed to 1 to 2. Three cases were considered to have "HELLP" syndrome comprising haemolysis, elevated liver enzymes, and low platelet count. Adult respiratory distress syndrome (ARDS) accounted for seven 'pulmonary' deaths and in another four it was thought to have been present. In one case, circulatory overload lead to fatal pulmonary oedema.

Substandard Care

Care was considered to be substandard in 24 of the 27 cases (89%). The cause was attributed to the patient herself in one, to the GP in four cases, all five of which received further substandard care in hospital. In one case both the woman and the GP contributed to substandard care. In two of the cases where the GP was involved, expert domiciliary assistance should have been called for eclampsia. In another case where the GP was not actually called, the ambulance service, apparently unaware of her pregnancy, took a woman who had convulsed to an Accident and Emergency Unit whereupon there were further inadequacies in the management of her eclampsia. In the remaining 17 cases the hospital obstetric team alone was considered responsible.

Patient Responsibility

An older grand multipara refused all antenatal care. She was seen at 27 weeks gestation with obvious fulminating pre-eclampsia, refused admission and later the same day had a fit at home. When admitted without the GP having called the Flying Squad, she reluctantly agreed to Caesarean section and was initially looked after postpartum in the labour ward due to a shortage of ITU beds. She died later in the ITU of another hospital. Autopsy was refused. The baby survived. The assessors felt that the shortage of ITU beds precluded adequate immediate postpartum care and may have contributed to the fatal outcome.

General Practitioner Responsibility

In two of the five cases involving a GP there was failure to refer in one and late referral in two others.

In the first, the blood pressure was much higher at 34 weeks gestation than at booking, there was proteinuria and fetal growth retardation. The patient was admitted "fortuitously" because of gastro-intestinal symptoms one week later, but had a fit two hours after admission before any urine testing or careful observation of blood pressure had been made. Caesarean section was performed the same evening, but overnight her care was substandard. Extra fluid was given postpartum to "chase a low urine output" and a CVP line was said to be "not working". The following morning she was transferred to an ITU where she died ten days later from ARDS.

In the second case the GP saw the patient at 25 weeks gestation with a blood pressure of 160/90mm Hg, having been 120/60mm Hg at the booking clinic. The hypertension persisted and she was only referred to hospital 25 days later, when her blood pressure on admission was 150/100mm Hg with proteinuria (+) and oedema. Elective Caesarean section was carried out 15 days later, but she died of ARDS postpartum. There was delay in GP referral and delay in delivery in the hope of obtaining a more mature fetus. At delivery marked ascites was noted, DIC had already developed, followed by ARDS which was the cause of death 32 days later.

In the third case a woman developed hypertension and subsequently proteinuria +++ and gross oedema over a period of several days. She was seen by three GPs during this period but when admission to hospital was eventually recommended she initially refused admission. Subsequently she had an emergency CS at 34 weeks gestation but succumbed to intracerebral haemorrhage.

In another case appropriate expert assistance should have been called as there was a history of a possible convulsion earlier in the day.

The patient was said to be conscious with a blood pressure of 140/90mm Hg when she left home accompanied only by her husband but she had a fit en route and on admission 45 minutes later her blood pressure was 160/120mm Hg. She had suffered placental abruption and DIC and died of cerebral oedema two days later. Even after admission the blood pressure was not adequately controlled and there was delay in getting the patient delivered.

Consultant Unit Responsibility

In 17 cases the Consultant Obstetric Unit alone was considered responsible for the substandard care. In these cases three factors were evident:

a. Delay in making clinical decisions.

b. Delay in Consultant involvement.

c. Inappropriate intrapartum and postpartum management, particularly blood pressure control.

In many cases more than one of these often interrelated factors operated.

a. *Delay in making Clinical Decision*

In this respect delay adversely affected the outcome principally in three ways.

First, there was often delay in instituting adequate treatment for significant hypertension soon after admission.

Second, there were examples of delay in getting the patient delivered soon enough, in some cases the reason being to gain fetal maturity. This factor may have operated in six cases with fatal results. The following is a typical example.

A patient with a booking BP of 120/70mm Hg had a triplet pregnancy. She was admitted at 28 weeks gestation with a blood pressure of 140/100mm Hg, proteinuria (+) and marked oedema (++).

Four days later the blood pressure was 160/115mm Hg for which she was given a single intra-muscular dose of hydralazine. Attempts were made to prolong the pregnancy even further by using labetalol. The proteinuria persisted and the platelet count fell 11 days later. The proteinuria then increased markedly and 13 days after this she had a Caesarean section but died of severe haemorrhage in relation to DIC. The fetal gestation at delivery was 31 weeks and all three babies survived.

A third form of delayed clinical decision making was failure to deliver sufficiently early, labour being induced rather than carrying out immediate Caesarean section.

A primigravida in her thirties had a booking clinic blood pressure of 110/60mm Hg at 27 weeks gestation. Two weeks later her blood pressure was 140/110mm Hg and there was proteinuria (++++). As the cervix was "ripe" on her admission, labour was induced with vaginal prostaglandins. The blood pressure was poorly controlled in labour, which lasted 10 hours, during which she had an eclamptic fit. In the course of this she vomited and aspirated. It had been hoped an epidural would control her blood pressure. She had no other form of antihypertensive therapy in labour before the fit.

b. *Delay in Consultant Involvement*

There were seven cases where this factor operated. In five of these junior staff had clearly failed to recognise the significance of serious symptoms and signs leading to late involvement of the consultant.

The following case illustrates many of the foregoing points.

A multigravida, normotensive at booking was found at 26 weeks to have a blood pressure 160/100mm Hg with marked proteinuria (++). She was admitted the same evening and an SHO on his own initiative prescribed a slow release calcium channel blocking agent to be taken orally. Overnight the diastolic blood pressure ranged between 105 and 120mm Hg and she was prescribed simple analgesics for headaches and anti-emetics for nausea and vomiting. The headaches were eventually ascribed to sinusitis. Control of oral medication was difficult because of persistent vomiting. The same oral anti-hypertensive drug was repeated the following morning when she was seen by a different SHO and Registrar. As the diastolic blood pressure was still ranging between 100 and 130mm Hg it was suggested that she be seen by the Consultant in the afternoon. She had further anti-hypertensive therapy orally and when she was eventually seen by the Consultant 22 hours after admission she was very quickly transferred to a High Dependency Area and given a bolus of hydralazine intravenously followed by further oral anti-hypertensive therapy. Her blood pressure then fell steeply to 130/75mm Hg but the proteinuria increased. Overnight blood pressure surveillance was reduced because it was disturbing sleep. By the following morning she was found unconscious and died soon after. Autopsy showed brain stem infarction, hypertensive encephalopathy and the renal changes of severe pre-eclampsia.

In the seven cases where consultant involvement was judged to be "too little" or "too late" or both, the majority had been handled by junior staff for too long with failure to appreciate the serious underlying nature of the case. Often when the Consultant became involved the situation was virtually irretrievable. This suggests a continuing lack of awareness of the potential seriousness of seemingly mild symptoms and signs and the treacherous nature of pre-eclampsia and imminent eclampsia, and a persisting failure by consultants to alert junior medical staff to these dangers.

In this context two cases presented atypically in that in one referred to later in this chapter there was substantial hypertension with virtually no proteinuria. In the other proteinuria was very marked but the blood pressure remained low initially, suddenly increasing dramatically. In both circumstances the intensity of care was relaxed and monitoring became inadequate because of the atypical presentation.

c. *Inappropriate Management*

Intrapartum Management. In two cases there was clearly inadequate control of hypertension in labour and in three others epidural analgesia alone was relied upon as in the case previously referred.

Postpartum Management. Unsatisfactory post partum care still accounts for a large part of the mortality from the hypertensive disorders of pregnancy, as was evident in 12 cases. Many of them had already had substandard antepartum or intrapartum care. The principal causes were:

a. Failure to have a clear cut strategy for postpartum blood pressure and proteinuria monitoring in patients who have been in any way hypertensive before delivery, and particularly during labour.

b. Symptoms such as headache, vomiting and epigastric pain being considered trivial and inadequately treated because the true cause was not recognised.

c. Poor communication between medical and midwifery staff.

As an example of the first, a patient with a twin pregnancy remained normal in most respects till 36 weeks gestation when she developed proteinuria, hypertension and marked oedema. Six g/24 hours of proteinuria was evident two days after admission. Labour was managed with epidural analgesia only, during which the blood pressure rose to 150/105mm Hg. As the blood pressure was "satisfactory" post delivery no specific care was given overnight apart from prochlorperazine for nausea along with simple analgesics for headache. Thirty-two hours after delivery the blood pressure was 150/95mm Hg, she felt "rotten", had blurred vision and was vomiting. She was therefore seen by an SHO, but no action was taken. Two hours after this, with a diastolic blood pressure of 115mm Hg, she suddenly collapsed. Despite immediate treatment with hydralazine and labetalol, she died in an ITU three days later of cerebral haemorrhage with an associated HELLP syndrome.

In another case the patient had had a Caesarean section for severe hypertension with a trace of proteinuria. On the third post partum day the blood pressure was still 170/110mm Hg, although there was now no proteinuria. She was seen by junior staff who felt that "impending eclampsia was only a remote possibility", no clear instructions were given and opiates alone were used for "sedation" and blood pressure control. She was later found unconscious and died soon afterwards.

The cause of death in this case ascertained at autopsy was pulmonary oedema in relation to severe pre eclampsia and possible overtransfusion. There had been very poor communication between medical and midwifery staff throughout.

Other aspects of substandard care

Reference to a Regional centre was made in eight of the cases, three being actually transferred for management of the pre-eclampsia. In two an opinion about management was sought and in one a transfer was made to ensure access to adequate paediatric facilities. Two other cases were transferred only after serious deterioration requiring intensive care had already taken place. The BEST survey may help to elucidate this important aspect of care which has been referred to and strongly advised in previous Reports but apparently not yet widely implemented.

Ergometrine, either alone or in combination with Syntometrine, was used in five cases where blood pressure was already substantially raised in labour and in two it may have been the only factor producing a very sharp blood pressure rise postpartum leading to the fatal outcome.

Organisation of care was poor and was severely criticised by assessors in three cases. In two cases there was poor communication concerning postpartum care between midwifery and medical staff and in the other ITU facilities were inadequate.

Other Clinical features

As 20 of the cases died in Intensive Therapy Units there is clearly now major involvement of anaesthetic staff in such cases.

Seven cases had ARDS confidently diagnosed and in four there was possible ARDS. DIC was evident in 15 of the 27 cases and in three, HELLP syndrome was present.

In two cases very severe pre-eclampsia developed between antenatal visits, the interval between which accorded with acceptable standards of present day practice. Thus if any future strategy for antenatal care is to mean fewer antenatal visits for apparently low risk cases there will continue to be some who may suddenly deteriorate within less than one or two weeks, as occurred in those cases.

The most commonly used anti-hypertensive agent in the cases reported here was labetalol to control hypertension, with hydralazine and diazepam used in the acute situation. Chlormethiazole, phenytoin and nifedipine were each used only once and in different cases.

Pathology

Autopsies were performed in 22 of the 27 cases; of these 12 were in women with pre-eclampsia, and 10 with eclampsia. Only 10 autopsies could be regarded as having been of a high standard.

Of the 12 unsatisfactory autopsies, three were of a poor standard, lacking organ weight, and two of these were without any histology. The other nine cases were regarded as unsatisfactory because of inadequate histology reports, although in other respects some of these autopsies were satisfactory. Because hypertensive disorders of pregnancy, particularly severe pre-eclampsia and eclampsia, produce typical lesions in the liver and kidney it is important to study the histology of both these organs in order to support the clinical diagnosis. Many pathologists did not do so. In one case with clinical pre-eclampsia the severe liver disorder was actually found to be acute fatty liver of pregnancy when the histology was reviewed by the regional pathology assessor.

All the autopsies in this group of cases were performed by experienced pathologists, the majority (16) on the instruction of the Coroner or Procurator Fiscal.

The quality of the autopsy was not influenced by the source of the request, in that seven of the 15 Coroner/Fiscal reports were "very satisfactory" as were two of the four where a clinician had requested the autopsy.

In two autopsies the requesting authority was not clear.

Five cases had no autopsy. Two of these were considered to have developed ARDS and each died in an Intensive Therapy Unit (ITU) while two died in a neuro-surgical unit following intracranial haemorrhage. The fifth, an eclamptic, was thought to have cerebral oedema on CT scan. She also died in an ITU.

Comment

A marked fall in the number of deaths from hypertensive disorders of pregnancy was noted in England and Wales between the triennia 1979-1981 and 1982-1984. Unfortunately there has been no such fall in the last two UK triennia which is very disappointing, particularly as the underlying causes of death and aspects of substandard care remain substantially unchanged.

Anti-hypertensive regimens, although often applied too late appear to have become more standardised. Unfortunately the obstetricians involved in many of the cases herewith reported often seem to have been either confident of their care, later considered by the assessors to be substandard, or to have been apparently taken unawares, particularly when informed late. This happened many times because junior medical and midwifery staff had underestimated the significance of symptoms and signs. This suggests a continuing lack of awareness of the importance of strategies for antepartum, intrapartum and particularly postpartum care of the patient with any degree of raised blood pressure, with or without proteinuria. The hypertensive disorders of pregnancy seem still not to be taken seriously enough in many cases. The reason for the persistence of this adverse aspect of care despite repeated pleas in these Reports is not clear and is worrying. Again the BEST survey may give further help in this respect.

Obstetric Units must impress on all staff from the first day of appointment, the treacherous nature and lethal potential of the hypertensive disorders of pregnancy. They must put in place careful and stringent strategies for monitoring the symptoms and signs of the hypertensive disorders of pregnancy particularly postpartum.

A recent survey covering 95% of UK obstetric units showed that nine percent still have no eclampsia protocol. This requires to be rectified immediately.

The system of referral to Regional Centres for advice and/or assistance does not yet appear to have become systematised despite the strong case made for this in previous reports.

Only two Regions had a clearly defined Regional policy. Only 76% of units had an ITU on the same site. Reference: Hibbard B M and Milner D G. Reports on Confidential Enquiries into Maternal Deaths. An audit of previous recommendations. (Accepted for publication early in 1994 in Health Trends.)

Any product containing ergometrine should not normally be used in hypertensive women.

Epidural analgesia in labour should not be relied upon by itself to control blood pressure in pre-eclampsia. This has been stated before in these Reports.

Attempts to secure a more mature fetus must not blind obstetricians to the dangers of a disease process which may be inexorably progressive despite blood pressure readings apparently controlled by antihypertensive drugs.

Women who have fits outside hospital require immediate expert attention before transfer. In the past hospital based "Flying Squads" have been available but cannot provide an optimal service. It is more appropriate that primary response in such cases should be by ambulance paramedics trained in cardiopulmonary resuscitation and the immediate management of obstetric complications. In England and Wales there is now a nationally agreed syllabus for training paramedics in the management of obstetric emergencies. (see chapter 17)

We endorse the recommendations of the Joint Committee of the Royal Colleges and Ambulance Service that the primary response for domiciliary emergencies such as eclampsia should be by ambulance paramedics trained in cardiopulmonary resuscitation and the immediate management of obstetric complications.

Obstetricians should keep themselves informed about patients who are transferred to ITUs and on occasion to neuro-surgical units to ensure wherever possible that should death occur an autopsy is arranged. In this way diagnoses will be more accurate and lessons learned.

CHAPTER 3

Antepartum and Postpartum Haemorrhage

Summary

Of the 22 deaths directly due to antepartum and postpartum haemorrhage, five were due to placenta praevia, five to placental abruption, one to coagulation failure associated with intrauterine death and eleven to postpartum haemorrhage. There were no *Late* deaths. Care was substandard in 14 of the 22 deaths. In addition to these 22 *Direct* deaths bleeding was implicated in four other deaths which are dealt with in their relevant chapters. The number of *Direct* deaths from haemorrhage has more than doubled since 1985–87.

Only deaths due to haemorrhage from the genital tract are included here. Deaths due to haemorrhage from other sites are considered in the appropriate chapters.

In 1988–90 there were 22 *Direct* deaths from haemorrhage with a mortality rate of 9.2 per million maternities, compared with 4.5 per million in 1985–87. There were no *Late* deaths. Of these 22 *Direct* deaths eleven were caused by antepartum haemorrhage (ICD 641) — five by placenta praevia, five by placental abruption and one by intrauterine death — and eleven by post-partum haemorrhage (ICD 666). Care was considered substandard in 14, compared with seven of the ten deaths in 1985–7 and six of the nine in 1982–4.

Table 3.1 *Number of deaths from haemorrhage and rates per million maternities, England and Wales 1973–90 compared with United Kingdom 1985–90*

	Placenta praevia	Placental abruption	Postpartum haemorrhage	Total	Rate per million maternities
England & Wales					
1973–75	2	6	13	21	10.9
1976–78	2	6	16	24	13.7
1979–81	3	2	9	14	7.3
1982–84	2	2	3	7	3.5
1985–87	0	4	6	10	5.0
1988–90	5	5+1*	10	21	10.1
United Kingdom					
1985–87	0	4	6	10	4.5
1988–90	5	5+1*	11	22	9.3

*The additional case was of antepartum haemorrhage in labour consequent on fetal death in utero.

Table 3.1 shows the number of *Direct* deaths from haemorrhage by cause and the death rate per million maternities in the five triennia from 1973–75 in England and Wales and in the two triennia from 1985–87 in the United Kingdom (UK). In addition to the 22 *Direct* deaths discussed in this chapter there were four (including one *Late* death) from other causes in which bleeding played a significant part. Two of these women had not attended for antenatal care, and two had bleeding problems after developing hypertension. These four cases are considered in their relevant chapters.

An older woman who had concealed her pregnancy died at home after bleeding from a major degree of placenta praevia. Autopsy showed that the cause of death was pulmonary embolism. The case is counted in Chapter 4.

A grossly obese woman was apparently unaware that she was pregnant. She had a previous classical Caesarean section and died of haemorrhage from spontaneous rupture of the uterus at term. The case is counted in Chapter 8.

A young woman with a triplet pregnancy developed hypertension at 28 weeks' gestation and was delivered by Caesarean section. She developed disseminated intravascular coagulation and despite further surgical interventions for bleeding she died at six days. The case is counted in Chapter 2.

A young primigravida developed hypertension at 34 weeks gestation and was delivered by Caesarean section. She developed a large haematoma, underwent laparotomy and was transferred to an Intensive Therapy Unit (ITU) where she developed respiratory problems and died 61 days later. This case is counted in Chapter 15.

The death rate by age per million maternities given in Table 3.2 indicates an increased risk with age, particularly for those aged 35 and over.

Table 3.2 *The number of deaths from haemorrhage, and death rates per million maternities by age from haemorrhage, United Kingdom 1988–90*

Age (years)	Maternities	Number of deaths	Rate per million
Under 20	193,130	0	0.0
20–24	631,861	2	3.1
25–29	836,433	6	7.2
30–34	499,873	8	16.2
35–39	167,543	4	23.9
40+	31,469	2	63.6
All ages	2,360,309	22	9.3

Seven of the nineteen women were of Afro-Caribbean or Asian origin, three of whom died from placenta praevia and two from placental abruption.

Placenta praevia

Five maternal deaths were caused directly by placenta praevia. Three of the five patients were over 30. One of the five was primigravid, three had had one baby before and one had two previous deliveries. Three of the five women had at least one previous Caesarean section.

Care was substandard in all five cases of placenta praevia. In one case this was because the woman had not attended at all for antenatal care: the first her doctor knew of her pregnancy was when she was found dead at home from haemorrhage. In the other four cases placenta praevia had been diagnosed and an elective Caesarean section had been carried out by an obstetric registrar without direct consultant supervision. In one case (an older hypertensive primigravida with a major degree of placenta praevia) the anaesthetist was also a registrar.

Successive editions of this Report have recommended that elective or emergency Caesarean section for placenta praevia should be performed or directly supervised by a consultant obstetrician. It is disappointing that after the 1985-87 triennium, during which no deaths associated with placenta praevia occurred, this advice now seems to be in danger of being forgotten.

Placental abruption

Five maternal deaths were due directly to placental abruption. Three of the women were over 30. One woman had no previous pregnancies, another had one previous miscarriage and the others had one, two and five previous deliveries.

Care was substandard in four cases of placental abruption, but in two this was because the woman had no access to medical help. One woman concealed her pregnancy and in the other case the medical staff were denied access to the woman by her violent husband. In two cases aspects of the medical care were judged to be substandard:

> An older multigravida presented at about 20 weeks of pregnancy having just arrived in the United Kingdom. Neither she nor any of her family spoke English and communication had to be via an interpreter. She had at least five previous pregnancies. Her haemoglobin fell to 8.3g/dl during the pregnancy and the hospital asked the GP to investigate and treat this anaemia. Folic acid deficiency and iron deficiency were diagnosed. The GP prescribed various oral iron preparations and later added folic acid suspen-

sion. She apparently did not take her medication because of gastro-intestinal symptoms. She was admitted at term with acute placental abruption. Her haemoglobin on admission was 5g/dl: she had a gross clotting deficiency and very poor urine output. She was delivered by vacuum extraction eight hours after admission and had an uncontrollable postpartum haemorrhage from which she died within two hours despite emergency hysterectomy.

During the antenatal period her anaemia should have been treated more energetically by the hospital. During labour there should have been more prompt treatment of the clotting disorder and a consultant anaesthetist should have been involved at an earlier stage, as the anaesthetic senior registrar was reluctant to insert a CVP line in the presence of the clotting disorder. A CVP line could have been inserted for instance, via a cubital vein.

In the other case in which care was sub-standard, abruptio placentae occurred, Caesarean section was carried out by a senior house officer and post-operative monitoring was sub-standard. This case is discussed further in Chapter 9.

In the fifth case of abruptio placentae the final cause of death was respiratory and hepato-renal failure associated with disseminated intravascular coagulation, due to a number of possible factors of which one was placental abruption:

> A primigravid patient was admitted with an intrauterine death and a tense uterus. Labour was stimulated with intravenous Syntocinon and the interval between starting the infusion and delivery was 21½ hours. During labour she became pyrexial and towards the end of labour clotting studies became abnormal. At delivery, 300 mls blood loss was recorded, with the presence of a retroplacental clot. Twenty minutes later the patient collapsed with unrecordable blood pressure. She was transferred to ITU. She had metabolic acidosis and developed DIC and pulmonary oedema. Liver enlargement was noted and she was transferred to a Liver Failure Unit, where a working diagnosis of septicaemia complicated by DIC was made. Amniotic fluid embolism was also considered. She died next day despite intensive treatment. Postmortem needle biopsy of the liver showed severe necrosis: permission for autopsy was refused.

Although there were flaws in the resuscitation in this case it is doubtful if her care could be regarded as substandard.

Intrauterine death

> A woman booked at 25 weeks gestation and intrauterine death was diagnosed. A coagulation screen was normal and prostaglandins

were used to induce labour. Vaginal bleeding began and six hours after induction she collapsed. Repeat coagulation screen showed no fibrinogen. She died within 80 minutes of collapse. The size of the fetus was appropriate for 22 weeks gestation. There was no evidence of amniotic fluid embolism at autopsy.

In Table 3.2 this case is added to the total of deaths from abruptio placentae.

Postpartum haemorrhage

Most of the cases of antepartum haemorrhage also involved postpartum haemorrhage but these deaths have not been counted as due directly to postpartum haemorrhage. Eleven deaths were due directly to postpartum haemorrhage in the absence of antepartum haemorrhage.

Seven of the eleven women were aged over thirty. None was of high parity. The past obstetric histories of the eleven were: no previous pregnancy (4), one miscarriage (2), one termination (1), one previous normal delivery (1), one previous Caesarean section (1), two previous Caesarean sections (1), unknown (1).

Caesarean section

Postpartum haemorrhage followed Caesarean section in four cases. In three the indication for operation was pre-eclampsia and DIC occurred, probably as a result of the pre-eclampsia. One of these cases involved a 91-unit blood transfusion.

> A chronic paranoid schizophrenic developed signs of pre-eclampsia (details not provided) at 38 weeks gestation. In late pregnancy she had refused any investigation or monitoring. Labour was induced but cervical dilatation ceased at 9cm. She had to be restrained for induction of anaesthesia for Caesarean section. After the operation 60mg depixol was given. Respiratory arrest occurred, and during resuscitation there was massive postpartum haemorrhage due to DIC.

There were insufficient staff available on a busy delivery suite at night to give this patient satisfactory care.

> A primigravida in her thirties developed fulminating pre-eclampsia. There was proteinuria for four weeks before her admission but her GP did not refer her to hospital. On admission she was ill but was not seen by a consultant. Caesarean section was carried out by a registrar. After the operation she had anuria and developed pulmonary oedema, liver failure and renal failure. She developed septicaemia and DIC, and haemorrhage could not be controlled despite hysterectomy.

Care was substandard at all stages of this case. The GP failed to refer her to hospital with early signs of pre-eclampsia. She was not seen by a consultant after admission. Caesarean section in such an ill patient should have been carried out by a more senior doctor. Treatment after delivery was inadequate.

A case in which intraperitoneal bleeding was followed by cardiac arrest after inadequate observation on the postnatal ward is discussed in Chapter 9.

Instrumental delivery

Postpartum haemorrhage followed forceps delivery in three cases, and vacuum extraction in one case.

> In an induced labour acute fetal distress occurred and delivery was effected by forceps when the cervix was 7cm dilated. Postpartum haemorrhage was complicated by DIC, and back-up facilities were inadequate.

It is not clear whether the haemorrhage resulted from trauma or DIC, but during investigation of the haemorrhage bleeding appeared to be coming from a vessel in the cervix. Instrumental delivery before full cervical dilatation is extremely dangerous.

> A patient had had a previous Caesarean section for APH. The obstetrician applied Kielland's forceps nine minutes after the start of the second stage of labour: the indication for forceps delivery is not clear. Slow but steady postpartum bleeding occurred and the severity of blood loss was not recognised until too late.

> A primigravida had a forceps delivery for fetal distress. Soon afterwards her blood pressure fell and moderate vaginal bleeding occurred. The SHO phoned the consultant and took the patient to theatre for suturing of vaginal lacerations. This was unsuccessful and by the time the consultant arrived DIC had developed. In spite of intensive treatment, including internal iliac artery ligation, the patient died eleven hours after delivery.

These two cases illustrate the danger of not recognising the severity of postpartum haemorrhage. In one case the blood loss was steady but undramatic and in the other case the SHO failed to appreciate that the blood was not clotting. Suturing of the vagina in a case of traumatic postpartum haemorrhage complicated by hypotension should have been carried out by a more senior doctor than an SHO.

> A primigravida was booked for an isolated GP unit in spite of being asthmatic. After spontaneous labour second stage delay occurred and vacuum extraction was carried out. During delivery of the placenta acute uterine inversion occurred. The uterus was replaced immediately but incompletely. Adequate resuscitation

facilities were not available. Transfer to the nearest intensive care unit took one and three-quarter hours. Blood loss was estimated at 3000ml and she suffered cardiac arrest.

Asthma attacks can occur at any time during pregnancy, including labour, and this patient should have been booked for a consultant unit. Blood should have been available. Uterine inversion is a rare complication that requires immediate skilled treatment including facilities for anaesthesia and resuscitation. These are not available in isolated GP units.

Spontaneous delivery

There was only one death from PPH following spontaneous delivery but there were other complicating factors.

> In a woman who had had two previous Caesarean sections labour was induced at 28 weeks because of intrauterine fetal death. The placenta was retained and was abnormally adherent, possibly to the uterine scar. Haemorrhage occurred and hysterectomy was carried out three hours later. (Subsequently it was found that one ureter had been doubly ligated at hysterectomy). The patient developed DIC, adult respiratory distress syndrome and renal failure and was transferred to a larger hospital for haemofiltration.

Transfer to the larger hospital was delayed and should have occurred earlier.

Coagulation failure

Disseminated intravascular coagulation is always a risk with obstetric haemorrhage, even before blood transfusion is begun. Coagulation failure was a feature of eleven cases, and in four other cases there was inadequate information to tell whether coagulation failure had occurred. Definite coagulation failure complicated three cases of placenta praevia; at least three of the five cases of placental abruption (information was inadequate in two); the case of intrauterine fetal death and four of the five cases of PPH.

Substandard Care

Some aspect of care was substandard in 14 of the 22 cases reported here, and the standard of care was doubtful in five of the others. In two cases this was the fault of the woman, for not reporting her pregnancy, and in another case a violent husband prevented staff from attending his wife. In the four cases of placenta praevia who underwent Caesarean section, the operation was carried out by an unsupervised registrar. These operations should be performed or supervised directly by a consultant. Other aspects of substandard care were failure to recognise clotting defects (three cases) and failure to insert a CVP line (four cases).

Pathology

Of the 22 cases where death was due to antepartum or postpartum haemorrhage, autopsies were performed on all but one. In eight the autopsy report was of a high standard, in six it was adequate but in seven the autopsy report was inadequate or missing.

There is a need for clinicians to liaise with the pathologists so that useful autopsy reports can be produced. For detailed comments on the pathology of these cases see the section on Antepartum and Postpartum Haemorrhagein Chapter 16.

Comment

It is disappointing that the number of deaths from haemorrhage has almost doubled since the last Report, as has the number in which care was considered substandard. As severe obstetric haemorrhage becomes less frequent, obstetricians may have become less vigilant and less experienced in treating these life-threatening emergencies. The cases described here suggest that both these factors may be operating. Diminished vigilance by consultant obstetricians allowed four of the cases of placenta praevia to be operated on by registrars.

Placenta praevia, particularly when associated with a previous uterine scar, may be associated with uncontrollable haemorrhage at delivery and hysterectomy may be necessary: the presence of a consultant at operation is essential.

Deaths from traumatic postpartum haemorrhage can also occur when vigilance is relaxed. The rule that full cervical dilatation is a prerequisite for forceps delivery must not be flouted and the suturing of vaginal lacerations in theatre in a hypotensive patient should not be left to an SHO.

Attention is drawn to the importance of maternal age. With the marked fall in the numbers of highly parous women in recent years it has become clear that maternal age is an important risk factor for haemorrhage even among women of low parity.

In the treatment of haemorrhage, accurate estimation of blood loss is vital, as is prompt recognition and treatment of clotting disorders, with the early involvement of a consultant haematologist. Resuscitation should involve a consultant anaesthetist. Attention is drawn to the use of adequately sized intravenous cannulae and the monitoring of central venous pressure.

Attention is also drawn to the guidelines for the management of massive obstetric haemorrhage, published in the previous Report and annexed to this chapter.

A recent survey[1] of consultant obstetric units in the United Kingdom showed that 86% of units are now on DGH sites (range from 63% in Scotland to 88% in England). 82% had a protocol for the management of massive haemorrhage (range from 24% in Northern Ireland to 89% in England). 87% have a blood bank on site (range from 54% in Scotland to 79% in England). Regional figures are also provided in the article1.

The number of units now lacking the desirable facilities discussed here is relatively small and rectification of the deficiencies should have a high priority with the providers of obstetric care. Standards should be monitored by the purchasers as well as the providers and by the Royal College of Obstetricians and Gynaecologists through its mechanism for the recognition of training posts.

The isolation of the maternity unit from resuscitation facilities including cardiac arrest teams was a factor in two of the deaths. The place of isolated units and GP units is still a subject of discussion. If death from haemorrhage occurs once in 100,000 deliveries a GP unit may encounter such a tragedy less than once in a century. In this triennium no death from postpartum haemorrhage occurred in a healthy woman who had a spontaneous vaginal delivery, and the key to maintaining safety in GP units is rigorous exclusion of women with risk factors.

Reference

1 Hibbard B M and Milner D G. Reports on Confidential Enquiries into Maternal Deaths. An audit of previous recommendations. *Health Trends* (Accepted for publication early 1994)

Annexe to Chapter 3

Revised guidelines for the management of massive obstetric haemorrhage

Summon all the extra staff required, including obstetricians, midwives and nurses. *In particular the duty anaesthetic registrar should be contacted immediately as in most obstetric units the anaesthetists will take over the management of the fluid replacement.* Alert the haematologists and the blood transfusion service who should be asked to be fully involved in the case as soon as possible. Make sure porters are available and warned that they will be required at short notice.

At least 20ml of blood should be taken (or an amount agreed by the local departments concerned) for blood grouping, cross matching and relevant coagulation studies. A minimum of six units of blood should be ordered. When plasma-reduced blood is used, additional colloid is likely to be necessary if more than 40% blood volume is replaced. Modified fluid gelatin or hydroxyethylstarch solutions are perfectly satisfactory at this stage of fluid replacement. Human albumin solution (4.5%) combined with red cells and crystalloids may be best if massive haemorrhage continues. Dextrans are not recommended.

All patients should be given blood of their own group as soon as possible. If the blood bank is informed of the urgency, ABO and Rh D compatible blood can usually be made available on an emergency basis soon after receipt of the cross match sample. Only if transfusion must be given immediately should uncrossmatched Group O Rh D negative blood be used.

At least two peripheral infusion lines should be set up using cannulae of not less than 14 gauge. Central venous pressure (CVP) monitoring should immediately be set up since it helps ensure that therapy is safely controlled. Central venous pressure should be continuously displayed and a display of intra-arterial pressure is also extremely useful.

Facilities for the measurement and display of CVP, intra-arterial pressure, ECG, heart rate, blood gases and acid base status should be available to all consultant obstetric units.

Regular haemoglobin or haematocrit assessment can be helpful in the control of blood and fluid therapy, but restoration of normovolaemia is the first priority. Platelet counts and coagulation studies should be performed as a guide to the presence of haemostatic failure including disseminated intravascular coagulation (DIC). Abnormal results will show the necessity for replacement therapy (e.g. Fresh Frozen Plasma(FFP); Cryoprecipitate; or Platelet Concentrates).

Rapid administration of fluids intravenously should be achieved by use of a compression cuff on the plastic bag. Martin's pumps and chambers for hand pumping do not give blood fast enough in exsanguinated patients and should not be used.

Blood must be administered through blood warming equipment.

Blood filtration is not usually necessary and may delay blood transfusion.

Additional calcium administration is rarely required and only if there is evidence of a Ca deficiency. 10% calcium chloride is preferable to calcium gluconate.

All patients with prolonged or massive haemorrhage require proper monitoring of pulse rate, blood pressure, CVP, blood gases, acid base status and urinary output as well as dedicated continuing care by the midwifery, nursing and medical staff. Early consideration should be given to the advantages of transfer to an intensive therapy unit.

More detailed reading

1. Guidelines for transfusion for massive blood loss. *Standard Haematology Practice*. Blackwell Scientific Publications. 1991. Pages 198–206.
2. Hewitt P E and Machin S J. Massive Blood Transfusion. *Brit. Med. J.* 1990; **300:** 107–109.

CHAPTER 4

Thrombosis and Thromboembolism

Summary

There were 33 deaths from thrombosis and/or thromboembolism counted in this chapter: 24 from pulmonary embolism and 9 from cerebral thrombosis. In addition, four *Late* deaths from pulmonary embolism are counted in Chapter 15.

There were 13 antepartum deaths (including 3 following ectopic gestation) and 11 postpartum deaths from pulmonary embolism. Of the antepartum deaths, seven occurred before the 20th week and 11 before the 33rd week: the youngest of these women was aged 28. In five cases symptoms of thrombosis were inadequately treated.

Of the 11 postpartum deaths, four of the women were aged over 35 and four weighed over 96kg. Eight of the eleven deaths followed Caesarean section. In three cases symptoms suggestive of thrombosis had not been investigated.

Of the nine deaths from cerebral thrombosis, four were antepartum and five were postpartum.

Deaths from thromboembolism and cerebral thrombosis are counted as *Direct* causes of maternal death and are discussed in this chapter. Twenty four deaths were coded as pulmonary embolism (ICD 673.2). In addition eight cases are mentioned in this chapter but counted in other chapters.

> Two women had ovarian cancer. An older obese woman died before being seen in the antenatal clinic at eight weeks gestation: at autopsy she had extensive ovarian cancer and the case is counted in Chapter 14. The other woman was a Late death and is counted in chapter 15.
>
> A young insulin dependent diabetic woman developed hypertension and was delivered by Caesarean section. There were problems with endotracheal intubation. She suffered cardiac arrest and died four and a half weeks later in ITU. The case is counted in Chapter 9.
>
> Five *Late* deaths are counted in Chapter 15. Four of these *Late* deaths were directly related to obstetric causes (pulmonary embolism) and one *Late* death from cerebral infarction was thought to be unrelated to obstetric causes. Of the four deaths from pulmonary embolism, one occurred 56 days after termination of preg-

nancy with prostaglandins for missed abortion, and one was an obese multigravida with sickle trait who had a massive pulmonary embolism a few weeks after a Caesarean section. Another obese woman collapsed 80 days after a Caesarean section. The fourth was an obese woman in her thirties who had a normal delivery after induction of labour at 42 weeks gestation. She was readmitted with deep venous thrombosis 12 days after delivery. A ten day course of heparin and support stockings were prescribed. Subsequently cough and breathlessness were inadequately treated and she was readmitted with pulmonary embolism 42 days after delivery. She died four days later.

The *Fortuitous* death was also a *Late* death from cerebral infarction four months after a normal delivery. She had been recommenced on oral contraception by her GP at the time of her postnatal visit.

Pulmonary Embolism

The twenty-four deaths from pulmonary embolism in the UK in 1985–90 are compared with those for England and Wales for the period 1973–90 in Table 4.1. Following an increase in antepartum embolic deaths in the previous triennium there has been a fall in this triennium. The number of deaths after vaginal delivery is the lowest ever. The number of deaths from pulmonary embolism after Caesarean section has not fallen during the last twenty years. However as the number of Caesarean sections has risen steadily the incidence of pulmonary embolism following CS has fallen.

Table 4.1 *Deaths from pulmonary embolism, England and Wales 1973–87, compared with United Kingdom 1985–90*

	Deaths after abortion or ectopic pregnancy	Deaths during pregnancy	Deaths during labour	Deaths after vaginal delivery	Deaths Total after Caesarean section
England and Wales					
1973–75	3	14	0	13	636
1976–78	2	14	0	20	945
1979–81	5	11	1	4	728
1982–84	4	9	0	4	1,229
1985–87	1	16	0	5	325
1988–90	3*	10	0	2	823
United Kingdom					
1985–87	1	16	0	6	730
1988–90	3*	10	0	3	824

* Three deaths after ectopic pregnancy (on days 1, 5 and 8). In addition there was one late death 56 days after mid-trimester prostaglandin termination of pregnancy for fetal abnormality.

A comparison of the interval between delivery and pulmonary embolism following vaginal deliveries and Caesarean section is shown in Table 4.2. In the present triennium two thirds of deaths after Caesarean section occurred within 14 days of delivery, whereas two thirds of deaths after vaginal delivery occurred after 14 days.

Table 4.2 *Interval between delivery and pulmonary embolism following vaginal delivery and Caesarean section, United Kingdom 1985–90*

	up to 7 days	8–14 days	15–42 days	Total
Vaginal delivery	0	3	6	9
Caesarean section	5	5	5	15

Antepartum

An analysis of the period of gestation of all the antepartum deaths in 1988–90 is as follows:

Up to 12 weeks	5 deaths (including 3 following ectopic gestation)
13–27 weeks	3 deaths
28 weeks to term	5 deaths

The salient features of these thirteen deaths are given in Table 4.3. Five of the thirteen cases occurred in the first eight weeks of pregnancy, underlining the importance (noted in the last Report) of considering this diagnosis even in early pregnancy. The youngest of the women was aged 28 and five were aged over 35. Five of the women had complained of symptoms of thromboembolism before death: three had leg pain, one chest pain and one breathlessness. Two were being treated with heparin.

Postpartum

There were eleven postpartum deaths due to pulmonary embolism and brief details are given in Table 4.4. Eight of the women had Caesarean section: three of these weighed around 100kg, two were aged 38 and 40, and the remaining three (aged 25, 27 and 31) had no other identified predisposing factors. Of the three women who had a normal delivery, one was aged 40, one weighed 133kg, and the third had a twin pregnancy after four previous pregnancies.

Age

The effect of age is tabulated in Table 4.5, which clearly shows the steady increase in risk with increasing maternal age, particularly over the age of 40.

Table 4.3 *Antepartum venous thromboembolism*

Age	Gestation in weeks	Features noted
Under 35	4?	Moderately obese, on mini-pill. Ruptured ectopic pregnancy: emergency laparotomy — ITU. Died 5 days later.
	5	Sickle-cell trait. IUCD. Ectopic pregnancy: salpingectomy. Died one day after operation.
	5	7th pregnancy. Spoke no English. Suspected ectopic, but pregnancy intrauterine.
	8	Mildly obese. IUCD. Ectopic pregnancy: salpingo-oophorectomy. Died 8 days later.
	21	Admitted to medical ward with breathlessness: treated for chest infection: died 24h later.
	30	Hereditary spherocytosis. Admitted with anaemia. Had leg pain and breathlessness.
	32	Wt 114kg. Mental handicap.
	35	Haemoptysis, coma & hemiparesis before delivery: died in ITU 4 days after CS.
Over 35	8	Previous DVT. Sterilisation reversal & failed IVF. On heparin for suspected DVT.
	16	Attended GP with chest pain: reassured. Tachycardia 140/min at AN clinic: ECG normal.
	19	Calf pain at 13 weeks: venogram normal. Heparin given in prophylactic dose.
	28	Concealed pregnancy. No antenatal care. Previous concealed pregnancies.
	30	Wt 88kg. Bed rest for wt loss. Leg oedema

IUCD = Intrauterine contraceptive device
IVF = In vitro fertilisation
AN = Antenatal
ECG = Electrocardiogram

Substandard Care

Care was considered substandard in six cases of pulmonary thromboem-bolism — three antenatal and three postpartum cases. In one of the ante-natal cases care was substandard because the woman had concealed the fact that she was pregnant and had no antenatal care.

Table 4.4 *Postpartum venous thromboembolism*

Age	Post-partum day	Mode of delivery	Features
Under 35	5	CS	Failed forceps. No ITU on site.
	9	CS	Wt 101kg. Went home well on day 7.
	10	CS	Post-op pyrexia. Breathless on day 7.
	16	ND	Para 4. Twins. Collapsed at delivery
	24	CS	Wt 101kg. In hospital 13 days postpartum
Over 35	1	CS	Uncomplicated CS. No other cause.
	1	CS	?Silent DVT before labour.
	2	CS	Wt 97kg. Pre-CS bed rest.
	13	CSS	low to mobilise. Unexplained pyrexia on day 9.
	15	ND	Emboli dislodged at laparotomy for retroperitoneal-haematoma.
	37	ND	Wt 133kg. Attended GP with tightness in legs 3 weeks postpartum, and with cough and breathlessness 2 days before death.

Table 4.5 *Maternal deaths due to pulmonary embolism by age, UK 1985–90.*

Age (years)	Maternities (thousands)	Number of deaths	Rate per million
Under 25	1,662.8	3	1.8
25–29	1,614.1	19	11.8
30–34	937.5	12	12.8
35–39	319.6	13	40.7
40 and over	58.1	7	120.5
All ages	4,592.1	54	12.0

An older parous woman in early pregnancy called out her GP because of chest pain. There were no physical signs and she was reassured that it was musculoskeletal. When she was seen later at the antenatal clinic she gave a history of breathlessness at times over the last month and she was noted to have a tachycardia of 140/minute. An ECG was normal. Her haemoglobin was 9.3gm/dl and the tachycardia was thought to be due to anaemia. She was admitted for investigation of anaemia and died four days later. Autopsy showed pelvic deep vein thrombosis and pulmonary embolus.

The hospital clinic had no notification of her episode of chest pain. No ventilation/perfusion scan was carried out. She was not seen by either a consultant physician or a consultant obstetrician. Greater awareness is required of the possibility of thromboembolism in an older woman, even in early pregnancy.

> An older woman complained of calf pain in early pregnancy. A venogram was carried out and was reported as normal. Subcutaneous heparin was given for only a week. At 18 weeks gestation she was admitted to hospital with spontaneous rupture of the membranes and two days later she had a fainting attack which was diagnosed clinically as pulmonary embolism. She was transferred to a medical ward and was heparinised but died less than an hour later. The presumptive diagnosis was pulmonary embolus but, surprisingly, no autopsy was carried out.

The venogram, which was reported by a clinical assistant in radiology, was wrongly interpreted and therefore inadequate treatment was given.

> A primigravid woman had forceps applied by a registrar while two-fifths of the fetal head were palpable per abdomen. Caesarean section was then carried out for failed forceps by the same registrar: disimpaction of the fetal head was difficult. Four days later the patient collapsed with cyanosis, tachycardia and hypotension. She was transferred to the intensive therapy unit (ITU) in another hospital, where despite exemplary care she died within a few hours. Postmortem examination showed a large mass of embolus in the main pulmonary trunk. Transfer to the ITU took one hour fifteen minutes.

More senior involvement in the delivery might not have made any difference to the outcome but would have been desirable. The fact that the maternity unit was in a different hospital from the ITU is also regrettable.

> A older woman who was grossly obese complained to her GP about tightness in her legs three and a half weeks after delivery. A fortnight later she attended the surgery complaining of breathlessness and cough. She was examined by one of the partners and no abnormality was detected. Two days later she died of pulmonary embolism.

> A woman booked for elective Caesarean section was admitted with spontaneous rupture of the membranes. Caesarean section was carried out but there is no evidence of any prophylaxis against deep venous thrombosis. During the puerperium she had a low-grade pyrexia and on the seventh day she complained of faintness, giddiness and shortness of breath. She had similar symptoms on the eighth day. On the tenth day she died of a massive pulmonary embolus.

In both these cases care was considered substandard because of failure to heed clear warnings of pulmonary embolism during the puerperium, even though both women were at risk — one because of her weight, the other because of the Caesarean section.

Pathology

Of the 24 Direct deaths, autopsies were performed on 22. In the two cases without autopsy, pulmonary embolectomy was performed on one and, in another a venogram, initially reported as negative for deep vein thrombosis of the legs was subsequently interpreted as positive.

Detailed discussion of the pathology of the cases may be found in the Pulmonary Thromboembolism section of Chapter 16.

Cerebral thrombosis

There were nine cases of cerebral thrombosis, compared with two cases in the triennium 1985–87. This increase may be accounted for by better diagnosis with CT scanning. Of the nine cases, four occurred during pregnancy (age range 19–34) and five in the puerperium (age range 25–36). Other details are given in Tables 4.6 and 4.7.

Table 4.6 *Antenatal cerebral thrombosis*

Gestation in weeks	Summary
8	Found collapsed in bathroom. CT scan showed middle cerebral artery thrombosis. Died after 2 days. autopsy confirmed diagnosis.
13	Headaches in early pregnancy. Left-sided weakness at 13 weeks. CT scan showed large right parietal haemorrhagic infarct. Died one day later. Autopsy confirmed superior sagittal sinus thrombosis.
20	Collapsed at 20 weeks, died 7 days later. CT scan showed sagittal sinus thrombosis.
26	Previous DVT. Heparinised. Convulsions at 26 weeks. CT scan showed cerebral infarction. Died after 3 days. No autopsy.

CT   = computerised tomography
DVT = deep venous thrombosis

Pathology

Cerebral venous thrombosis: There were six deaths attributed to cerebral venous sinus thrombosis and a further four attributed to cerebral infarction of which one was a Late death. Autopsies were performed on five of the six cases of venous sinus thrombosis. Histological examination of the brain was performed on only one case. In two of these five cases thrombosis of the superior sagittal sinus was demonstrated. In a third case streptokinase had been injected into the superior sagittal sinus and thrombus was demonstrated in the right lateral (transverse) and sigmoid sinuses, extending into the internal jugular vein. In the remaining two cases in which autopsy was performed thrombosis was described in the superficial veins of the brain. In one of these there was meningitis but the superior sagittal sinus was not examined. In the other case, although venous sinus thrombosis was reported there was no detail of the site of this thrombosis.

Table 4.7 *Postpartum cerebral thrombosis*

Day	Del	Summary
5	CS	Previous CS x2 and previous DVT. Elective CS. Heparinised. Collapse on day 5, died four days later. CT showed internal carotid occlusion.
12	VE	Sagittal sinus thrombosis due to meningitis. Initially mistaken for puerperal psychosis.
15	CS	Eight previous pregnancies. Smoker. Elective CS. Collapsed and died on day 7. Intracranial haemorrhage with lateral sinus thrombosis.
15	ND	Obese, hypertensive. Labour induced at 38 weeks. Normal delivery, normal puerperium until day 8 — headache, vomiting, confusion, followed by collapse. Died 2 days later. Autopsy showed cerebral and pelvic venous thrombosis.
19	CS	Known epileptic, with history of DVT. Heparinised in pregnancy. "Pre-eclampsia" at 30 weeks. Two fits after admission, thought to be eclamptic. CS. Heparin stopped. DVT. Re-heparinised fully for 4 days, then prophylactic dose. CVA at day 15. Died 3 days later. Autopsy showed sagittal sinus thrombosis.

CS	=	Caesarean section
CT	=	computerised tomography
CVA	=	cerebrovascular accident
DVT	=	deep vein thrombosis
ND	=	normal delivery
VE	=	vacuum extraction

In the case which did not come to autopsy CT scan during life gave a diagnosis of superior sagittal sinus thrombosis.

Cerebral infarction: Only one of the four cases diagnosed as cerebral infarction came to autopsy. In this case there was infarction associated with left middle cerebral artery thrombosis. Two of the remaining cases were receiving heparin because of a preceding deep vein thrombosis in the legs. CT scan in one was described as showing cerebral infarction for which a cause could not be found. In the other, CT scan revealed thrombosis of the left internal carotid artery. The fourth case, a *Late* death, had a massive cerebral infarct, revealed by CT scan, in the distribution of the left middle cerebral artery four months after delivery of a term baby.

Comment

Thrombosis and thromboembolism remain a major cause of maternal death in the United Kingdom. Some deaths occur without warning, but many appear to be preventable by greater awareness of the significance of signs and symptoms of thromboembolism, and by greater vigilance in high-risk women. Attention is again drawn to the age of the women dying of pulmonary embolism: few were of high parity and it is clear that age itself is an important risk factor. Obesity is another factor that has been noted in previous Reports, although the exact risk cannot be quantified accurately because data are lacking on the number of obese women who delivered in the United Kingdom during the triennium.

It is clear that grossly overweight women are at increased risk of thromboembolism and deserve extra vigilance and counselling.

Table 4.8   *Risk factors for development of thromboembolism*

Previous thromboembolism
Obesity
Immobilisation
Operative delivery
Increasing Maternal age

All the deaths from antenatal pulmonary embolism occurred in women over the age of 28 and in some of these cases thrombosis had been suspected before the fatal embolism occurred. There must have been many cases during the triennium in which such symptoms were correctly treated, and it may seem a counsel of perfection to demand 100% accuracy in this diagnosis. Nevertheless, as pointed out in previous Reports, the dangers of anticoagulant treatment seem to have been exaggerated in the past.

Our recommendation remains that any woman who is pregnant or who has recently been pregnant and has a suspected deep vein thrombosis or pulmonary embolism should be given full anticoagulant therapy. In postpartum cases, a bilateral venogram and lung scan should be carried out within 24–48 hours.

Attention is drawn to the guidelines on thrombosis associated with pregnancy published by the Haemostasis and Thrombosis Task

Force.[1] These guidelines emphasise the need for accurate diagnosis, the usefulness of real time ultrasound and impedance plethysmography, and the safety of limited or, if necessary, full venography.

The advice given in the last Report on the diagnosis of thrombosis is repeated here:

> Whilst venograms are contraindicated in the first trimester of pregnancy, even though the uterus can be shielded off, they can certainly be used in the third, and possibly the second, trimester. Real time ultrasound scanning can be used in pregnancy even though it is unlikely to detect thrombus in the iliac veins because of the gravid uterus. In these circumstances it is unlikely that there will be significant thrombus in the iliac veins without there also being some in the femoral veins. A ventilation-perfusion isotope lung scan can be used for the diagnosis of pulmonary embolism as the radiation dose to the fetus [about 0.2 milliGrays] is low.

The estimated dose equivalent of a ventilation/perfusion scan is 1 milliSievert, which is approximately half a year's background radiation.

The fall in the number of deaths from pulmonary embolism after normal delivery is encouraging. It is possible that this fall is a consequence of the trend towards increased mobility during labour and earlier mobilisation after delivery. Two of the deaths after normal delivery in this triennium were in unusual cases — a patient with a retroperitoneal haematoma and a woman who weighed 133kg.

The number of deaths due to thromboembolism after Caesarean section has not changed over the years. Because numbers of Caesarean sections have increased, the rate of death from pulmonary embolism must have fallen but it appears that wider use of prophylactic anticoagulation or other methods of prophylasis in high-risk cases could reduce the risk still further. Obesity and increased age are again the two risk factors that recur in this Report as in previous Reports. It is also important to note that in two thirds of the cases death after Caesarean section occurred after the seventh post-partum day. This underlines the importance of GPs and midwives knowing which women are at high risk and reacting promptly to warning symptoms.

All those involved in the care of pregnant or recently pregnant women should consider pain in the leg, pain in the chest, or dypsnoea in an otherwise healthy woman to be due to thrombosis or pulmonary embolism until proved otherwise.

---

[1] Maternal and Neonatal Haemostasis Working Party of the Haemostasis and Thrombosis Task Force. "Guidelines on the prevention, investigation and management of thrombosis associated with pregnancy". *Journal of Clinical Pathology* 1993; **46**:489–496.

CHAPTER 5

Amniotic Fluid Embolism

Summary

There were eleven deaths due to amniotic fluid embolism in the United Kingdom (UK) in 1988–90 compared with nine in 1985–87. Seven were associated with induced labour and two with Caesarean section. None of the women was of high parity, and all were aged over 25.

Only deaths where autopsy provided histological evidence of amniotic fluid embolism (AFE) have been accepted for the UK reports for 1985–90.

There were eleven *Direct* deaths attributed to amniotic fluid embolism and classified under ICD 673.1. There was one death in which there was a clinical impression of amniotic fluid embolism without confirmation of the diagnosis at autopsy. In a further four cases the possibility of AFE had been considered but could not be confirmed because of inadequate autopsy information. The case is considered in Chapter 10. The deaths of four women who were found to have products of conception in the circulation were ascribed to other causes.

Age

Table 5.1 gives details of the age of the women with proven amniotic fluid embolism. The risk of this condition increases with age. In the present triennium, no case of amniotic fluid embolism occurred in a woman under the age of 25.

Table 5.1 *Maternal deaths from amniotic fluid embolism by age and estimated rates per million maternities, United Kingdom 1988–90*

Age (years)	Maternal deaths	Maternities (x1000)	Rate per million maternities
Under 25	0	825.0	–
25–29	6	836.4	7.2
30–34	4	499.9	8.0
35–39	0	167.5	–
40 and over	2	31.5	63.3
All ages	11	2,360.3	4.7

Parity

There is no association between amniotic fluid embolism and parity. None of the eleven patients was of high parity: six were nulliparae and two of these six had never been pregnant before. One had one previous delivery and each of the other four had had two term pregnancies.

Induction or augmentation of labour

Table 5.2 shows the number of cases in which prostaglandin or oxytocin had been given. Only two patients had gone into labour spontaneously, and one of those was a woman booked for elective Caesarean section because of two previous Caesarean sections. Six of the eleven patients had had prostaglandin pessaries. Of these six, three also received an intravenous infusion of oxytocin, three had artificial rupture of the membranes and one had both.

Table 5.2 *Clinical features of cases of amniotic fluid embolism*

Parity+ Early Pregnancy Loss	Complications ante partum	Induction/ augmentation of labour	Complications	
			intra partum	post partum
0+1	Diabetes	Elective CS		Collapse
2+1	Abnormal CTG	PG+ARM	Slow FH – CS	PPH
2+2	"Flu"	–	–	PPH
2+0	Prev CS (x2)	–	Slow FH – CS	PPH
2+0	Prev CS	PG	Seizure – FD	
0+1	Pre-eclampsia	PG+ARM+Synt	Collapse – CS	
1+0	Amniocentesis	PG+ARM	Collapse – CS	
0+1	Weight loss	PG+Synt	–	Collapse
0+0	Asthma / PE	PG+ARM	Collapse – CS	
0+3	Cervical cerclage	PG+Synt	Slow FH – CS	PPH
0+0	Twins / PE	CS at 32/52	–	Collapse

CTG	= cardiotocograph
CS	= Caesarean section
PE	= pre-eclampsia
PG	= prostaglandins for induction of labour
ARM	= artificial rupture of the membranes
Synt	= intravenous infusion of syntocin (oxytocin)
FH	= fetal heart rate
PPH	= postpartum haemorrhage
FD	= forceps delivery

A primigravid patient had weight loss at term and for this reason prostaglandin pessaries were inserted four days before labour was induced by artificial rupture of the membranes and oxytocin infusion. After a normal labour and delivery she developed a brisk postpartum haemorrhage. The doctor who repaired the episiotomy called the consultant but did not seem to appreciate that the blood was not clotting. The patient quickly collapsed.

Although the outcome may well not have been altered in this case, doctors should be alert to the possibility of amniotic fluid embolism if postpartum haemorrhage occurs without adequate explanation.

Mode of delivery

Two of the eleven patients had a normal delivery: one developed brisk postpartum haemorrhage soon after delivery and the other more slowly.

Of the nine women who underwent operative delivery, the indication in four cases was maternal collapse which was presumably the first sign of amniotic fluid embolism.

One patient had a forceps delivery minutes after a grand mal seizure, followed quickly by cardiac arrest.

Eight patients were delivered by Caesarean section. One Caesarean section was elective and another was carried out after failure of induction of labour for pre-eclampsia. Of the six emergency Caesarean sections, three were because of the sudden onset of fetal distress and three because of collapse of the mother.

Speed of collapse

In seven of the eleven cases the clinical presentation was of sudden collapse of the woman, either during or after labour. In five of these seven cases, death occurred within two and a half hours. In the other two cases the patient died later in an intensive therapy unit.

The clinical presentation in two of the remaining cases began with fetal distress, and maternal death occurred three and a half hours later in each case.

In the remaining two cases the onset of the condition was more insidious and the time course was slower. One of these is described in the section on "substandard care". In the other case care was not substandard.

> Before labour a woman had a flu-like illness with sore throat and during labour she was unwell. She had a normal delivery. The baby was ill for a week and had DIC, and a Group A haemolytic streptococcus was cultured. The mother had continuing blood loss and six hours after delivery she had torrential bleeding and pulmonary oedema. Tests showed DIC. The blood loss was controlled but she died twelve hours after delivery.

In the three cases in which death occurred within an hour of collapse there was no evidence of DIC, but in all cases in which death occurred more than two hours after collapse there was evidence of a coagulation disorder.

Substandard care

Amniotic fluid embolism is a condition with a high mortality, and treatment, however rapid and efficient, is often unsuccessful. Therefore clinical and administrative deficiencies revealed in these cases were frequently judged not to have affected the outcome. Nevertheless, in order to learn useful lessons, instances of substandard care are described.

> In a hospital which had a policy of not cross-matching blood before Caesarean section (unless there were special indications) there was a failure to have adequate blood and blood products available on the delivery unit. The operating department assistant was unfamiliar with the delivery unit and the anaesthetic registrar was a locum. Blood was not requested until after the end of the operation, when heavy blood loss had already occurred and the patient was already hypotensive. The obstetric team left theatre before the patient was moved to the recovery area (in spite of the patient having had 1.5L blood loss) and did not realise the speed of her deterioration.

> A heavy smoker had a Caesarean section in labour for fetal distress. There was difficulty in achieving haemostasis during closure of the abdomen, but the patient was sent to a postnatal ward rather than a high-dependency bed. She was shaking uncontrollably and wheezing but there was delay in appreciating the seriousness of the problem and respiratory problems were ignored because she was a heavy smoker. Three hours later excessive bleeding was noted through the wound and per vaginam and the blood was not clotting. The wound was re-explored and no bleeding point was found. DIC was diagnosed and treated but the patient was not transferred to an ITU. The maternity unit was an isolated building and the nearest ITU was 2–3 miles away. Neither this nor two other units contacted had any beds available. She died within 24 hours of delivery.

Failure to provide intensive therapy was judged to be substandard care, as was the lack of consultant involvement. The consultant anaesthetist was unobtainable and the consultant obstetrician gave telephone advice only.

> A woman who had one previous normal pregnancy, had labour induced at term with prostaglandins. The indication for induction is unclear. The membranes were ruptured artificially in labour and immediately afterwards acute fetal distress occurred, followed by

collapse of the woman. There was no resident anaesthetist in this hospital and the obstetrician had not alerted an anaesthetist to his plan to induce labour in a woman of short stature, aged over 40, with a high fetal head.

Failure to have an anaesthetist available was judged substandard care, although the presence of an anaesthetist is unlikely to have altered the outcome.

In another case the anaesthetist went to intubate the neonate. The anaesthetist should not have to interrupt supervision of the mother to intubate the baby.

Pathology

All cases came to autopsy and the diagnosis was confirmed by examination of the lungs. The presence of fetal squames was taken to confirm the diagnosis although it was not always clear whether special staining had been done.

More details are provided in Chapter 16.

Table 5.3 shows the number of deaths from histologically confirmed amniotic fluid embolism for England and Wales for the triennia 1973–90 compared with the UK for 1985–90.

Table 5.3 *Deaths from amniotic fluid embolism histologically confirmed and deaths suspected of being amniotic fluid embolism but not confirmed, England and Wales 1973–90, compared with United Kingdom 1985–90*

	Histologically confirmed cases	Suspected cases
England & Wales		
1973–75	14 (1)	7
1976–78	11	8
1979–81	18	6
1982–84	14 (1)	2
1985–87	9 (2)	1**
1988–90	11	1
United Kingdom		
1985–87*	9 (2)	2**
1988–90*	11 (1)	1**

The numbers in parentheses () are with amniotic fluid embolism present but death attributable to other Direct cause.

* United Kingdom data

** See text.

Comment

The number of maternal deaths from amniotic fluid embolism has risen in this triennium compared with 1985–7.

Some risk factors noted in previous Reports were again present in these cases – higher maternal age, and the use of oxytocic agents to induce or augment labour. However, other risk factors previously noted were not evident in this triennium – for example, none of the women was of high parity, and strong uterine contractions were not noted in any of the cases. Indeed, two of the women collapsed and died during elective Caesarean section.

The Report for 1985–87 drew attention to the use of a single bolus of Syntocinon or Syntometrine in the third stage of labour. This was not recorded among the eleven cases described here. In the present triennium seven of the eleven women received prostaglandins to induce labour. This suggests that the risk factor is not the type of oxytocic agent used, but the fact that uterine stimulation has occurred.

The definition of amniotic fluid embolism in this Report is based on the finding of amniotic squames in the lungs. It is possible that amniotic fluid can enter the circulation without a fatal outcome. The diagnostic criteria for amniotic fluid embolism and the understanding of its pathophysiology remain obscure.

It is again recommended that women dying after labour of causes other than suspected amniotic fluid embolism should have their lungs examined for amniotic squames to check whether the definition used in this chapter is correct.

The high mortality of amniotic fluid embolism may lead to a feeling that nothing can be done to treat the condition and little can be done to prevent it. Nevertheless, because the definition of the condition depends on postmortem findings it is not known how many women are successfully resuscitated after amniotic fluid embolism.

Extra vigilance is required in high risk women ie. older women in whom labour has been induced. If postpartum haemorrhage occurs in such a patient consultant staff should be promptly involved in the management and the patient should be rapidly transferred to an intensive therapy unit.

CHAPTER 6

Early Pregnancy Deaths

Summary

As in the previous Report all deaths from ectopic pregnancy and abortion have been considered under the heading Early Pregnancy Deaths. The total number of *Direct* and *Indirect* deaths related to ectopic pregnancy and abortion occurring in early pregnancy (defined as up to 28 weeks gestation) was 35 in this triennium compared with 36 deaths in the previous triennium. Thirty of these deaths were *Direct* obstetric deaths and five were *Indirect* deaths. There were 19 deaths from ectopic gestation with evidence of substandard care in seven, and 14 deaths following abortion, with substandard care in seven. In addition there were two women who had hydatidiform moles, mentioned below.

Twenty four deaths are counted in this chapter, and the 11 other deaths occurring in connection with early pregnancy are counted in other chapters: Chapter 4 (three cases), Chapter 12 (three cases), Chapter 11 (two cases) and Chapter 3 (one case). The other two cases concerned women who had hydatidiform moles: One developed sepsis and is counted in Chapter 7 and the other suffered profuse haemorrhage and died following a cerebro-vascular accident and is counted in Chapter 10.

Deaths from ectopic pregnancy and deaths from abortion are considered separately, abortion deaths being divided into deaths following spontaneous abortion and deaths following legal abortion.

Ectopic Pregnancy

There were 19 reported ectopic pregnancy deaths in this triennium which represents eight per cent of all *Direct* and *Indirect* maternal deaths. Fifteen of these deaths were a direct result of the rupture of the ectopic pregnancy and are counted in this chapter. All of the deaths occured in England and Wales and there were four more deaths than in the previous triennium. This is also more than double the rate of such deaths compared with the 1982 - 1984 triennium. Three women survived the initial event but died from subsequent pulmonary emboli and are counted in Chapter 4. A fourth woman died during status asthmaticus precipitated by the pain and shock of a ruptured ectopic pregnancy despite only 200ml blood loss, and is counted in Chapter 12.

Table 6.1 summarises the 35 early pregnancy deaths for this triennium.

Table 6.1 *Summary of Early Pregnancy Deaths UK 1988–1990*

Type of Case	Gestation in weeks	Sepsis +/– organism if known	Substandard Care	Chapter Number	*Direct/ Indirect*	ICD Code
Ectopic	?	–	Yes	6	*Direct*	633.1
Ectopic	8	–	Yes	6	*Direct*	633.1
Ectopic	?	–	No	6	*Direct*	633.1
Ectopic	?	–	N/S	6	*Direct*	633.1
TOP	7	–	Yes	6	*Direct*	635.9
SROM	17	+ Cl perfringens	Yes	6	*Direct*	658.4
SROM	24	+ E coli	N/S	6	*Direct*	658.0
Ectopic	7	–	No	6	*Direct*	633.9
Ectopic	8	–	No	6	*Direct*	633.9
Ectopic	7	–	No	6	*Direct*	633.9
Ectopic	10-14	–	Yes	6	*Direct*	633.9
Ectopic	7	–	Yes	6	*Direct*	633.1
Ectopic	?	–	Yes	6	*Direct*	633.9
SROM	23	+ E coli	Yes	6	*Direct*	639.0
SROM	23	+Staph. aureus E. coli	N/S	6	*Direct*	670.9
Ectopic	8	+ Gram-ve	No	6	*Direct*	633.1
Ectopic	?	–	No	6	*Direct*	633.1
Ectopic	?4	–	Yes	6	*Direct*	633.1
Ectopic	5	–	Yes	6	*Direct*	633.1
Ectopic	?	–	Yes	6	*Direct*	633.1
Ectopic	?	–	Yes	6	*Direct*	633.1
TOP	?	+ Gram-ve	Yes	6	*Direct*	635.0
TOP	19	–	Yes	6	*Direct*	639.2
SROM	19	+?Gram-ve	Yes	6	*Direct*	639.0
SROM	18+	+Haemolytic strep. Strep. millerii Bacteroides sp.	No	6	*Direct*	639.0
Ectopic	8	–	No	4	*Direct*	673.0
Ectopic	10	–	No	12	*Indirect*	493.9
Hydatidiform mole.	?	+Cl perfringens	No	7	*Direct*	639.0
SROM	22	–	N/S	12	*Indirect*	117.3
Hydatidiform mole.	17	–	Yes	10	*Direct*	630.0
Incomplete abortion	13	–	Yes	11	*Indirect*	745.4
Missed abortion	22	–	N/S	3	*Direct*	639.1
Ectopic	5	–	No	4	*Direct*	673.2
Ectopic	?4	–	No	4	*Direct*	673.2
Incomplete abortion	12	–	Yes	12	*Indirect*	637.3
SROM	?6	–	Yes	11	*Indirect*	648.6

TOP – Termination of Pregnancy
SROM – Spontaneous rupture of membranes
N/S – Not stated

There was also one other death which occurred nearly two years after a ruptured ectopic pregnancy during which hypoxic brain damage occurred and this case is described in Chapter 15.

Table 6.2 shows deaths from ectopic pregnancies and rates per million estimated pregnancies, in England and Wales. The figures given for total estimated pregnancies incorporate conception statistics based on date of conception (see Chapter 1). These data are not available routinely for Scotland and Northern Ireland. Numbers of ectopic pregnancies for 1988–1990 have been estimated from incomplete Hospital Episode Statistics for that period.

Table 6.2 *Deaths from ectopic pregnancies and rates per million estimated pregnancies, England and Wales 1973–90*

	Total estimated pregnancies in thousands	Ectopic pregnancies in thousands	Ectopic pregnancies per 10,000 pregnancies	Number of deaths	Deaths per million estimated pregnancies	Deaths per 1,000 ectopic pregnancies
England and Wales						
1973–75	2366.8	11.7**	49	19		1.6
1976–78	2275.8	11.6**	51	21		1.8
1979–81	2437.8	12.1**	50	20		1.7
1982–84	2426.9	14.4**	59	10*		0.7
1985–87	2650.9	N/A	N/A	11	4.1	N/A
1988–90	2886.9	24.0***	83	15	5.1	1.8

* There were 3 other deaths from anaesthetic
** HIPE – Hospital In-patient Enquriy
*** HES – Hospital Episode Statistics
N/A – Not available.

Substandard Care

Seven out of the 15 ectopic pregnancy deaths counted in this Chapter were thought to involve substandard care. They are described in detail.

Patient Responsibility

In two the actions of the patient were considered to have contributed to the outcome.

> A woman in her thirties was unwell for four days prior to her death but at first refused to allow a GP or an ambulance to be called. When she was severely ill the GP was called but the woman refused admission to hospital. When the doctor saw her next day she was in a state of irreversible hypovolaemic shock and suffered cardiac arrest on the journey to hospital. Immediately on admission she was operated on for the ruptured ectopic pregnancy but all attempts at resuscitation failed.

An older woman probably had not realised that she was pregnant. Two days before her death she had called a GP because of abdominal pain, vomiting and constipation. The doctor, who was deputising, diagnosed a possible intestinal obstruction and wanted to arrange admission to hospital but the woman refused. No doctor visited the following day. The next day her GP was called and found the woman dead. The autopsy showed a massive retroperitoneal haematoma arising from a ruptured ectopic pregnancy.

Although the latter patient was first involved by refusing admission to hospital, there was also medical responsibility in that no doctor visited her on the following day. This raises doubts about the mechanism of handover from the deputising doctor to the patient's own G.P.

Clinical Responsibility

In five cases there were substandard features in the clinical management.

An older woman had termination of a pregnancy in a private clinic after eight weeks of amenorrhoea. Three weeks later she was admitted as an emergency to an NHS hospital with vaginal bleeding and lower abdominal pain. A diagnosis of post-abortal infection was made and she was treated with antibiotics. Twelve hours later she collapsed and a ruptured tubal ectopic pregnancy was suspected. Whilst being prepared for transfer to theatre she had a fit and was found by the duty medical registrar to have no significant cardiac output. Resuscitation was commenced and six units of blood were rapidly transfused. The registrar performed an emergency laparotomy on the ward, during which the consultant arrived. The predominant cardiac state remained asystole and resuscitative measures were discontinued.

No histological evidence was available to confirm whether there had been an intrauterine pregnancy at the time of the termination. No scan was carried out on admission and no senior member of staff saw the woman following her admission with signs and symptoms which, although leading to a reasonable diagnosis of sepsis, could have alerted a more experienced clinician to the possibility of ectopic pregnancy.

A woman in her twenties was admitted to hospital in hypovolaemic shock and early laparotomy was carried out for a seven week tubal abortion. At laparotomy there was about one litre of blood in the peritoneal cavity and she was transfused with blood. On the day after operation she became pyrexial and developed a cough. Later, chest signs were detectable, with widespread crepitations. Ampicillin was started but on the following day her condition was poor and more active treatment was given with bronchodilators, a nebuliser and intravenous erythromycin. Hydrocortisone was also given and she was transferred to the Intensive Therapy Unit (ITU). A diagnosis of Adult Respiratory Distress Syndrome (ARDS) was made with an associated coagulopathy which was never totally corrected and in spite of all resuscitative measures she died 36 days later. At autopsy ARDS was confirmed and there was a large subcapsular haematoma in the liver containing one litre blood clot with an underlying hepatic adenoma. It was thought likely that this was a long standing lesion and that the large blood loss may have arisen from the adenoma.

The management of the ectopic pregnancy cannot be criticised but the management and supervision of the patient before, during and after surgery was considered to be less than ideal, with no CVP monitoring or blood gas measurements until much later in the management of the ARDS.

> A young woman had a curettage following what was considered to have been a spontaneous abortion after ten weeks of amenorrhoea. However very scanty secretory endometrium was obtained at operation and the pathologist reported no evidence of pregnancy. A month later she called her GP because of pain and diarrhoea of acute onset and was given general advice. She died suddenly a few hours later. At autopsy there was a ruptured ectopic pregnancy with associated intra-abdominal haemorrhage.

It appears that none of those involved in her care checked the histology report or took any action based on it. No follow up had been arranged.

> A woman who was a heavy smoker was admitted to hospital with lower abdominal pain and vomiting. A diagnosis of ectopic pregnancy was made and emergency laparotomy was carried out. She required transfusion. Afterwards she developed chest signs thought to be infective in origin and antibiotics, bronchodilators and physiotherapy were prescribed. She collapsed on the first post operative day and was resuscitated by the cardiac arrest team and transferred to the ITU. She failed to regain consciousness and was pronounced brain dead ten days later. At autopsy pulmonary oedema and diffuse swelling of the brain were found and the cause of death was given as hypoxic encephalopathy and cardio-respiratory arrest.

The patient was nursed in an isolation room and episodes of cyanosis were not investigated. Errors in control of the fluid balance occurred resulting in a positive balance of about four litres. Although she weighed less than 50kg she received 60mg papaveretum in eight hours and this was considered excessive. No senior anaesthetist was involved with her peri-operative care.

> A young woman in her first pregnancy was admitted to hospital with acute abdominal pain and shock. She was transferred to the operating theatre immediately and at laparotomy the experienced registrar noted a left ruptured ampullary pregnancy with

haemoperitoneum++. Although two units of group O Rh negative blood and four units of uncrossed matched whole blood of the patient's group were available before induction of anaesthesia, this was not given. Three to four litres of modified fluid gelatin were transfused. The cross matched blood was available about half an hour after the patient was taken to theatre. About an hour after the operation the woman collapsed with pulmonary oedema, unrecordable blood pressure and no palpable pulses. As continued bleeding could not be excluded as a cause of this post-operative collapse the senior registrar decided on a second laparotomy. On this occasion the senior registrar noted definite bleeding from a corpus luteum of the left ovary and performed an oophorectomy. There was about one litre of sero-sanguinous fluid in the abdomen. The patient was then admitted to ITU by which time she had received about 16 units of blood and four units of fresh frozen plasma in addition to three to four litres of modified fluid gelatin. Her CVP was 26cm/H2O, consistent with fluid overload or acute heart failure. She was ventilated but the following week her respiratory function progressively deteriorated due to ARDS. Eleven days after the original operation she was transferred to another hospital with a view to lung transplant but did not survive the journey.

In this case there was delay in initiating blood transfusion at her original admission. It was thought that such a severely shocked patient should have been given group O Rh negative or blood of her own group without waiting for a full cross match. No consultant anaesthetist was called and monitoring was considered to be inadequate in the early stages of her management. The autopsy report was thought to be inadequate. The major organs were not weighed and neither microbiology nor histology was done to confirm the diagnosis.

Pathology

Autopsies were performed on all 15 *Direct* deaths due to ectopic pregnancy. In ten of these the report was satisfactory but in five it was inadequate. In one of the latter cases only the cause of death due to a ruptured tubal pregnancy was given, this diagnosis was later confirmed by the Regional Pathology Assessor who was able to examine histologically one block from the isthmus of the tube. In only three of the 15 autopsies was there adequate histology.

Comment

Ectopic pregnancy remains a major diagnostic challenge and an important contributor to maternal deaths. Where the diagnosis is in question, the involvement of an experienced clinician at an early stage is essential.

We again emphasise that the most important contribution to reducing the risk of death from ectopic pregnancy is an awareness by medical attendants that in any woman of reproductive age, an ectopic pregnancy may be the cause of a lower abdominal pain particularly when of sudden onset. The previous Report also emphasised important aspects of management which are repeated here.

When a woman presents with unexplained abdominal pain with or without vaginal bleeding she should not be allowed home until every means available has been used to exclude an ectopic pregnancy. The ready availability of beta-hCG kits for the detection of early pregnancy means that general practitioners in the home or surgery can easily make a diagnosis at an early stage of pregnancy. Vaginal examination is also essential to determine whether there is localised tenderness, or a palpable appendage mass. If there is any doubt, referral to hospital is preferable to a "wait and see" policy. Laparoscopy remains the cornerstone for investigating the possibility of an ectopic pregnancy and this should be done on any woman found to have a positive pregnancy test with an empty uterine cavity on ultrasound scan. Alternatively, if the pain persists for more than 24 hours despite a negative beta-hCG pregnancy test, then a laparoscopy should be done.

Ultrasound scanning makes an important contribution to the detection of an ectopic pregnancy. It is essential that an experienced sonographer should be asked to do the scan and unsupervised occasional sonographers should be discouraged.

Two of these deaths resulted from lack of treatment because the women refused admission to hospital. Although it is the right of any person to decline treatment nevertheless doctors must give adequate counselling and advice where the potential seriousness of the diagnosis is realised.

Both inadequate resuscitative measures and over transfusion leading to pulmonary oedema occurred in cases described here. ARDS is increasingly recognised as a complication of haemorrhage. Early diagnosis is essential for effective treatment and appropriate protocols should be available in all ITUs.

Aspects of the anaesthetist's contribution to resuscitation and monitoring are highlighted. Involvement of senior experienced anaesthetists is imperative, with early adequate transfusion of blood and careful monitoring using CVP lines to avoid over transfusion.

The already severely ill, collapsed patient is a diagnostic challenge and the anaesthetist, gynaecologist, ITU physician and pathologist must cooperate in planning management.

Abortion

In this section of the chapter deaths related to both legal and spontaneous abortion are considered. Although there were no deaths associated with illegal abortion, it is disappointing to note there were three *Direct* deaths from legal termination.

Table 6.3 contains data on abortion deaths for succeeding triennia in England and Wales from 1973, and for the United Kingdom since 1985. "Estimated pregnancies" includes conception data based on date of conception, see Chapter 1, and is not available for Scotland and Northern Ireland.

Table 6.3   *Direct abortion deaths in the triennial reports 1973-1990 by type of abortion per million maternities and rates per million estimated pregnancies.*

	Spontaneous	Legal	Illegal	Unspecified	Total	Rates per million maternities	Rates per million estimated pregnancies
England & Wales							
1973–1975	4	13[1]	10	–	27	14.1	10.5
1976–1978	2[2]	8[2]	4	–	14	8.0	6.0
1979–1981	6[5]	5[3]	1	2	14	1.3	5.5
1982–1984	4[4]	7[4]	0	–	11	5.8	4.4
1985–1987	4[6]	1[7]	0	–	5	2.5	1.9
1988–1990	4	3	0	–	7	3.0	2.0
United Kingdom							
1985–1987	5[6]	1[7]	0	–	6	2.7	N/A
1988–1990	6	3	0	–	9	4.0	N/A

[1]Does not include 1 anaesthetic death associated with legal abortion.

[2]Does not include 5 anaesthetic deaths, 4 associated with legal and 1 with spontaneous abortion.

[3]Does not include 1 anaesthetic death associated with legal abortion.

[4]Does not include 2 anaesthetic deaths, 1 associated with legal and 1 with spontaneous abortion.

[5]One other death is known to have followed a spontaneous abortion in the 1979–1981 triennium but it was reported too late to be included in the Enquiry.

[6]Includes one death from missed abortion.

[7]Does not include 1 unexplained death associated with legal abortion.

There were 14 deaths related to abortion of which nine are counted in this chapter. The other five deaths are counted elsewhere in this Report (Table 6.1 clarifies).

Spontaneous Abortion

Six women succumbed to post-abortion sepsis. Five other women, whose deaths followed spontaneous abortion, are counted in other chapters: Two women died subsequent to spontaneous abortion from pre-existing medical conditions, and are counted in Chapter 12. Two women with congenital cardiac disease aborted spontaneously in early pregnancy and are counted in Chapter 11. One patient had a missed abortion and died from haemorrhage following induction of labour. This case is counted and described in Chapter 3.

Post - abortion Sepsis

Six women developed septicaemia following spontaneous abortion compared with two in the previous triennium. Care was thought to have been substandard in four of the cases.

> A woman in her twenties had previously had a Caesarean section and a legal termination. She was admitted at 19 weeks gestation with spontaneous rupture of the membranes. On the following day she became pyrexial. After blood and vaginal cultures were taken, intravenous co-amoxiclav (Augmentin) was commenced. Spontaneous incomplete abortion ensued and two days after admission evacuation of retained products of conception was performed. At that stage she was hypotensive and hypothermic and had developed a coagulopathy. The SHO anaesthetist sought the help of the medical registrar and a CVP line was inserted. In spite of resuscitative measures she continued to deteriorate and died.

This case was managed by junior staff only and no senior member of staff was involved in the crucial early stages. Treatment in several areas was inappropriate and there was delay in her transfer to the ITU.

The following case illustrates the importance of ease of access to ITU.

> An older woman with a history of three previous spontaneous abortions and two elective Caesarean sections had been booked at 13 weeks for confinement in hospital. She was admitted at 23 weeks with bulging membranes. She was apyrexial and was treated conservatively. She became pyrexial on the day after admission and the membranes ruptured spontaneously with offensive amniotic fluid draining. Oral ampicillin was commenced but seven hours later when the temperature rose to 39°C, intravenous ampicillin was given. Within hours she collapsed and treatment for what was considered to be gram negative septicaemia was begun using hydrocortisone, metronidazole and gentamycin intravenously in addition to ampicillin. Abortion occurred one hour later but the placenta was retained and had to be removed under general anaesthesia. The woman's condition deteriorated after this and she died three hours later.

There was no available ITU, the nearest being four miles away and she was considered too ill for transfer.

> A young woman had spontaneous rupture of her membranes at 18 weeks gestation. She had previously had one full term normal delivery, two mid-trimester prostaglandin terminations of preg-

nancy, one of which was followed by pelvic sepsis with isolation of the gonococcus, and one first trimester incomplete abortion. Three days after spontaneous rupture of the membranes she developed a bacterial septicaemia and disseminated intravascular coagulation (DIC). Her further management included a hysterectomy and subsequent laparotomy to exclude a subphrenic abscess, but she developed ARDS and died just over a month after the initial event. Histology of the placenta confirmed severe chorioamnionitis and the uterus showed acute suppurative myometritis. Organisms isolated included Group F haemolytic streptococci, *Streptococcus millerii* and Bacteroides species.

An older parous woman had amniocentesis carried out at about 17 weeks gestation. On the night of the amniocentesis she became ill with vomiting, diarrhoea and gross haematuria. The next day she complained of abdominal pain and some bleeding and was admitted. She was found to be pyrexial with a distended abdomen and absent bowel sounds. She aborted spontaneously shortly after admission. Her condition deteriorated, with persistent hypotension, raised blood urea and grossly disturbed blood gases. Ventilation was attempted and she suffered a cardiac arrest. She was subsequently transferred to a renal unit and treated with broad spectrum antibiotics. She developed DIC with renal failure requiring intermittent renal dialysis. Nineteen days after the amniocentesis she had a laparotomy and hysterectomy performed. She continued to deteriorate and died two days later. There was no record of causal organisms, although the clinical picture was one of septicaemia. It was not clear whether the septicaemia was consequent upon the amniocentesis.

A young woman with a history of two previous spontaneous abortions was admitted to hospital at approximately 14 weeks gestation for insertion of a cervical suture. At 24 weeks the membranes ruptured and she was readmitted to hospital. Forty eight hours later she became pyrexial and intravenous co-amoxiclav was commenced. Within a few hours she collapsed and after resuscitation the suture was removed. DIC developed and she died in spite of resuscitation efforts. Clinically the picture was one of septicaemia but at autopsy DIC was confirmed and the possibility of amniotic fluid embolism was raised. Blood cultures were negative but E coli was cultured from the urine. Final assessment of histological specimens concluded that there was well established purulent placentitis. The cause of death was septic shock.

A young woman had previously had a spontaneous delivery at term. She was known to have sustained cervical damage from a previous extensive cone biopsy for carcinoma in situ. She was admitted at 25 weeks following premature rupture of the membranes, became pyrexial after 24 hours and antibiotic therapy was started. She deteriorated and syntocinon was commenced to stimulate contractions. This was unsuccessful and because of her condition hysterotomy was done. The patient collapsed and failed to respond to resuscitation. No autopsy was allowed. E coli and *Staphylococcus aureus* were cultured from placenta and uterus.

Legal Abortion

Three deaths are reported in this triennium from legal termination of pregnancy. In all three there was sub-standard care.

A young woman with poor social circumstances had a mid trimester termination by dilatation and evacuation after prostaglandin preparation of the cervix in the at a specialist private clinic. A large cervical tear was produced at subsequent dilatation and evacuation. She was returned to theatre for suture of the cervical tear. The extensiveness of the tear and the internal haemorrhage was not appreciated and the patient continued to deteriorate. Her death was confirmed soon after transfer to an NHS hospital.

This private hospital was approved by the Department of Health to undertake termination of pregnancy, but had not met all the requirements regarding consultant cover in this particular case.

A young multiparous woman had an mid trimester termination of pregnancy carried out in an NHS hospital. Vaginal prostaglandin was used for 48 hours followed by IV syntocinon for 48 hours. When no response was obtained extra-amniotic prostaglandin was commenced. Some 31 hours later abortion occurred and five hours after the abortion evacuation of retained products was carried out. Within 24 hours pyrexia ensued and ampicillin and metronidazole were commenced. Septic shock developed and in spite of intensive care the woman died five days later. At autopsy no evidence of trauma to the uterus was found.

This woman was at risk of infection because of the prolonged time involved (over five days) in attempting to abort her. No swabs were taken and no antibiotics were given at an early stage. When they were ultimately given it was considered that they were inadequate for such a situation.

A young woman with a complex social background concealed from the doctors the fact that she suffered from bronchial asthma occasionally requiring steroids. Following the pregnancy termination at seven weeks gestation she had a sudden and severe bronchospasm and failed to respond to resuscitative measures. The operation was carried out in a small private abortion hospital equipped for basic resuscitation only.

71

The woman failed to reveal her full medical history although questioned. Although immediate management was given by the experienced practitioners it was insufficient.

It is clearly impossible for small units to provide ITU facilities for resuscitation of complex cases but the Department of Health approval of private units does require and monitor emergency and referral arrangements.

Pathology

One of the three autopsies following death from legal abortion was unsatisfactory because no cultures were taken in spite of the clinical diagnosis of death from septic shock and there was no histological examination of the uterus. In only one of the three cases was there adequate histology.

Comment

Several cases yet again highlight the unfortunate tendency for junior staff to manage critical situations on their own without seeking help or even advice from senior medical staff. Not infrequently junior staff are hesitant to "trouble" their seniors and it must be emphasised yet again how short sighted is this policy. Protocols should emphasise, and re-emphasise, the necessity to inform consultants when any doubt exists as to the correct management of a case.

The use of an ITU at an early stage is also highlighted. In one case, the absence of an ITU was possibly crucial. This should never happen nowadays and it is to be hoped that there will be a swift end to the problem of split sites, which may involve a deficiency in emergency services.

It is disappointing to record three deaths from legal termination in this triennium compared with one in the previous triennium. Two of these terminations were carried out in the private sector and one in the NHS. The need for strict supervision of these cases, the awareness of potential problems, the competence of medical staff and the adequacy of available facilities are all highlighted.

CHAPTER 7

Genital Tract Sepsis Excluding Abortion

Summary

There were 17 deaths associated with genital tract sepsis in this triennium. This is a marked increase on the nine deaths which occured during the previous triennium. Seven of the deaths are counted in this chapter and the other ten are counted elsewhere in this Report. Eight of the latter ten cases were early pregnancy deaths and are counted in Chapter 6. One woman, admitted in labour with a 'flu like illness, is counted in Chapter 5. The other woman who had endotoxic shock following Caesarean section is counted in Chapter 10.

The number of deaths from sepsis from all causes including abortion and ectopic pregnancy, for succeeding England and Wales triennial reports since 1973 and for United Kingdom reports since 1985 is shown in Table 7.

Table 7.1 *Maternal deaths from genital tract sepsis including abortion and ectopic pregnancy with rates per million maternities, England and Wales 1973–1990, compared with United Kingdom 1985–1990*

	Sepsis after abortion	Sepsis after ectopic pregnancy	Puerperal sepsis	Sepsis after surgical procedures	Sepsis before or during labour	Total	Rate per million maternities
England & Wales							
1973–75	6	–	8	11	–	25	13.0
1976–78	7	–	6	9	–	22	12.6
1979–81	7	–	2	4	2	15	7.8
1982–84	3	–	–	1	1	5	2.7
1985–87	2§	1§	2	2	2	9	4.5
1988–90	5+§	1§	4*≠	5†	0	15	7.2
United Kingdom							
1985–97	2§	1§	2	2	2	9	4.0
1988–90	7+§	1§	4*≠	5†	0	17	7.2

* For 1988–1990 puerperal sepsis includes deaths following spontaneous vaginal delivery. Deaths following Caesarean section are included in Sepsis after Surgical Procedures.

+ Includes one case of sepsis after legal abortion.

§ These cases are counted in Chapter 6

≠ Includes one case counted in Chapter 5

† Includes one case counted in Chapter 10

The seven cases counted in this chapter have been divided into sepsis after surgery and sepsis after spontaneous delivery.

Sepsis After Surgery

Four women died from genital tract sepsis following surgery. Three of these women developed sepsis after Caesarean section, and there was one death from *Clostridium perfringens* infection following a dilatation and curettage (D&C). An additional case where septicaemia occurred following an elective Caesarean section in a young diabetic woman is counted in Chapter 10.

Details of the four cases are as follows:

> A multiparous woman died from necrotising fasciitis having been delivered by elective Caesarean section because of previous Caesarean sections. On the second post operative day she developed pain and abdominal distension with absent bowel sounds and was hypotensive and pyrexial. She had haematuria and diminished urine output. Blood was taken for culture and metronidazole and cephradine were commenced. The next day exploration of the wound was carried out and later that day the antibiotic regime was changed. Subsequently debridement of the anterior abdominal wall was required. Despite intensive treatment she continued to deteriorate and brain stem death was confirmed eleven days later. Coliforms and enterococci were grown on culture.

Necrotising fasciitis is extremely rare and exceptionally so in relation to Caesarean section. Whether prophylactic antibiotics would have altered the outcome is debatable but certainly this case raises again the question of the value of routine prophylactic antibiotics for Caesarean section.[1]

> A young primigravida with a persistent breech presentation was delivered by elective Caesarean section carried out under epidural anaesthesia. Her post operative progress seemed normal and the day before she died she was well with a slight pyrexia only. A mid-stream urine specimen (MSU) was sent for microbiological examination and she was commenced on cephalexin. She was found to be unconscious early on the fourth morning after the operation, and died despite attempts at resuscitation. At autopsy copious vomit was found in the larynx and trachea and there was necrotising ulceration of the uterine endometrium with purulent exudate. The cause of death was given as septicaemic shock with aspiration of vomit. No blood culture had been obtained and the MSU and culture of a post-mortem swab of the spleen were sterile.

> A woman in her thirties had an uneventful Caesarean section carried out at 41 weeks by a registrar, for hypertension and a breech

presentation. A wound infection developed requiring drainage and she became septicaemic. It is impossible to obtain full details as the case is sub judice. Endotoxic shock developed and in spite of apparently appropriate treatment, the patient died. The causative organisms were *Staphylococcus aureus* and *Enterobacter cloacae*.

An older woman presented with peri-menopausal bleeding and was investigated for possible uterine malignancy. The day after a D&C had been performed she developed pain and vomiting. Her condition deteriorated and she was returned to theatre for total hysterectomy and bilateral salpingo-oophorectomy. The naked eye appearance of the contents of the uterus suggested adenocarcinoma, but subsequent histology confirmed a hydatidiform mole. *Clostridium perfringens* was isolated. There was massive haemolysis and septicaemia from which she succumbed within a few hours.

Sepsis After Spontaneous Delivery

Three women died from sepsis of the genital tract following spontaneous delivery; two of these were young women who had concealed their pregnancies.

In addition there was a death of a woman who had a 'flu like illness with sore throat before labour, and was unwell during her labour. She subsequently developed DIC. Amniotic fluid embolism was diagnosed at autopsy. The baby was unwell and a Group A haemolytic streptococcus was cultured. This case is counted in Chapter 5.

A primigravida delivered spontaneously at 42 weeks gestation following induction of labour. She required a transfusion of two units of blood because of bleeding from a deep vaginal tear. Thirteen days later she was seen in a casualty department because of an ankle injury and a purpuric rash was noticed. Thrombocytopenia was confirmed and a haematologist was consulted. She was discharged home and was discovered dead in bed the next day. Autopsy showed endometritis and septicaemia, due to group A beta haemolytic streptococci, was given as the cause of death.

In this patient, who had been ill for a few days preceding her attendance at hospital, it was felt that further investigation of the thrombocytopenia should have been made.

A teenage primigravida concealed her pregnancy and had no antenatal care. She had a stillbirth at term. She became severely ill with puerperal sepsis and died shortly after admission to hospital in spite of resuscitative measures. The organisms cultured from the placenta were *Streptococcus millerii* and anaerobes.

A young primigravida concealed her pregnancy and went into labour at about 28 weeks gestation and delivered the baby at home. On admission to hospital she was severely ill and septic shock was diagnosed. In spite of resuscitation in ITU she died and autopsy confirmed septicaemia. There is no record of the organisms cultured.

Comment

These cases demonstrate once more that infection must never be underestimated and that it continues to be an important cause of maternal mortality. It must again be pointed out that sepsis can often be insidious in onset and progress in a fulminating way.

The question of prophylactic antibiotics must be continually under review. At present consensus opinion appears to be in favour of prophylactic antibiotics for Caesarean section.[1] When infection develops and the patient is systemically ill, urgent bacteriological specimens including blood culture must be obtained. It may be difficult to decide upon the appropriate antibiotic therapy and the advice of a microbiologist should always be sought.

Reference

1 Enkin M *et al.* *"Prophylactic antibiotics in association with Caesarean Section".* Chapter 73 *"Effective Care in Pregnancy and Childbirth."* Ed. Chalmers I, Enkin M, and Keirse MJNC. Oxford: OUP, 1989.

CHAPTER 8

Genital Tract Trauma

Summary

As in the previous report for the United Kingdom this chapter is concerned with maternal deaths directly due to genital tract trauma, including vaginal, cervical and uterine lacerations. There were three such deaths in this triennium. Two involved the body of the uterus, in the third there were lacerations of the vagina, cervix and possibly parametrium. Care was considered to be substandard in two.

Of the three *Direct* deaths due to genital tract trauma the uterus was ruptured in two, one through a classical Caesarean section scar, the other in association with a severe abruptio placentae. The third death followed uncontrolled bleeding from the birth canal after a forceps delivery.

Spontaneous Uterine Rupture

This occurred on two occasions.

> A very obese woman was in her second pregnancy; her first had terminated in a classical Caesarean section. She had a long psychiatric history with recurrent episodes of depression. She was not known to be pregnant; if she herself was aware of it she failed to declare it to anyone and had no antenatal supervision. At term she sustained a spontaneous rupture through the previous uterine scar before the onset of labour and died of massive intra-abdominal haemorrhage in the ambulance before reaching hospital. Autopsy confirmed massive intra-abdominal haemorrhage from a ruptured vertical uterine scar.

> A grande multipara sustained a severe abruptio placentae with intra-uterine fetal death at 37 weeks gestation. Artificial rupture of the membranes and low dose oxytocin stimulation was followed by spontaneous vaginal delivery. Persistent postpartum haemorrhage ensued associated with disseminated intravascular coagulation (DIC). The haemorrhage was uncontrollable despite vigorous intravenous therapy and eventual hysterectomy, laparotomy having revealed a longitudinal lateral rupture of the uterus. Recurrent ventricular fibrillation supervened and she died without recovering from anaesthesia.

The effect of oxytocin on the uterus of a highly parous woman damaged by accidental haemorrhage cannot be entirely discounted as a factor in the uterine rupture.

Traumatic Uterine Rupture

This occurred in one case following forceps delivery, with laceration of the upper vagina and cervix.

> A multiparous woman went into spontaneous labour at term and fetal distress developed. The cervix was thought to be fully dilated and she had a mid-cavity forceps delivery by the duty registrar. Subsequently there was persistent vaginal bleeding despite intravenous syntocinon and a well contracted uterus. An hour later she was examined by the consultant who found a three centimetre tear in the anterior lip of the cervix. Suture of this failed to control the bleeding. At laparotomy there was no intra-abdominal bleeding and it was thought that the haemorrhage was passing into the vagina from the lower segment. Hysterectomy was therefore performed. Marked oozing occurred from the pelvic tissues and the internal iliac arteries were ligated. During this procedure the left internal iliac vein was torn and the bleeding increased. There was now evidence of DIC, and the assistance of a vascular surgeon was obtained. As the bleeding could not be stopped by sutures the pelvic cavity was packed and the abdomen closed. The patient was then transferred to the intensive therapy unit but despite massive intravenous therapy her condition deteriorated and she died about eight hours after delivery. Autopsy disclosed a partially sutured vaginal tear which was apparently the source of the initial bleeding.

Pathology

In all three cases autopsies were performed and these were considered adequate in two and of high standard in the third. In two cases hysterectomy had been performed in an attempt to control bleeding. The pathologist ensured that the excised specimens were examined and revealed transmural tears, one through a Caesarean section scar. In the case where the internal iliac vein was torn and massive bleeding occurred, the pathologist failed to demonstrate the trauma to this large vessel. In the third case the uterus was examined in situ at autopsy. In only one of these cases was there a histological report and in this case histology was limited to the uterus. Postmortem histology is an important part of the investigation of spontaneous uterine rupture and failure to examine the uterus histologically in two of these cases is considered substandard.

Comment

The reduction from six to three deaths due to genital tract trauma in this triennium compared with 1985–87 is welcome; nevertheless substandard factors were considered to be present in two and possibly associated with the use of syntocinon in the third. The death due to haemorrhage after forceps delivery might have been avoided had the extent of the vaginal vault laceration been appreciated and the wound adequately sutured at an early stage.

CHAPTER 9

Deaths Associated with Anaesthesia

Summary

There were four deaths considered to be directly due to anaesthesia in this triennium. In addition there was one *Late* death (counted in Chapter 15) which was directly due to anaesthesia. One of the *Direct* deaths was due to problems with the tracheal tube, the second was associated with the inappropriate treatment of hypotension during a spinal anaesthetic and the third was due to substandard postoperative care. The fourth death and the *Late* death were due to aspiration of gastric contents.

There were an additional ten deaths in which it was considered that anaesthesia contributed to the death. Two of these patients died as a result of haemorrhage. Anaesthesia contributed to the death of two other patients who had pre-existing respiratory disease. The remaining six deaths were associated with substandard postoperative care.

Forty four of the 238 *Direct* and *Indirect* maternal deaths in this triennium (18.5%) were due to the Adult Respiratory Distress Syndrome (ARDS) or to associated complications. Eighteen of these deaths (41%) occurred in patients who had a hypertensive disorder of pregnancy. This topic is discussed in an annexe to this Chapter.

In the 1988–90 triennium there were 15 deaths associated with anaesthesia. Four of these were directly attributable to the anaesthetic. There was also one death directly due to anaesthesia which is classified as a *Late* death (Chapter 15). In another ten patients anaesthesia was considered to have contributed to the death. Deaths have again been classified as ICD 668 ("Complications of the administration of anaesthetic or other sedation in labour and delivery"). Table 9.1 shows the deaths directly attributable to anaesthesia in the triennia from 1973 to 1990. The marked decrease in *Direct* deaths seen in the last triennium has been continued.

Table 9.1 *Deaths directly associated with anaesthesia (excluding Late deaths), estimated rate per million maternities and percentage of Direct maternal deaths England and Wales 1973–90, compared with United Kingdom 1985–90*

		Number of deaths directly associated with anaesthesia	Rate per million pregnancies/ maternities	% of Direct maternal deaths
England and Wales	1973–75	27	10.5	11.9
	1976–78	27	12.1	12.4
	1979–81	22	8.7	12.4
	1982–84	18	7.2	13.0
	1985–87	5	2.4	4.1
	1988–90	3	1.4	2.3
United Kingdom	1985–87	6	1.9	4.3
	1988–90	4	1.7	2.7

Deaths directly due to anaesthesia

Table 9.2 summarises the four deaths and the one *Late* death directly due to anaesthesia. One death was due to a problem with the tracheal tube, a second to inappropriate treatment of hypotension after a spinal anaesthetic and a third to substandard postoperative care. The fourth death and the *Late* death were considered to be due to aspiration of gastric contents.

Table 9.2 *Deaths directly attributable to anaesthesia: procedures for which anaesthesia was given, indications for operation and cause of death*

Operation	Indication	Cause of death
Emergency planned Caesarean section	Pre-eclampsia and fetal distress	Hypoxia due to tracheal tube problem
Incision and marsupialisation of Bartholin's abscess		Pulmonary oedema after spinal anaesthetic
Emergency planned Caesarean section	Prolonged labour	Postoperative hypoxia and hypotension
Emergency unplanned Caesarean section	Failed trial of labour	Presumed aspiration of gastric contents
Late death		
Intended Caesarean section: forceps delivery	Delay in second stage	Aspiration of gastric contents

(For Caesarean section classification see Chapter 13)

The patient required an emergency planned Caesarean section for pre-eclampsia. During a previous Caesarean section for the same indication the anaesthetist had noted that the "inflation pressure was high, suggesting pulmonary oedema". On this occasion the anaesthetist (an SHO with 10 month's experience) attempted to give a spinal anaesthetic, but this was abandoned at the patient's request. Anaesthesia was induced with thiopentone and suxamethonium after pre-oxygenation and the application of cricoid pressure but the trachea could not be intubated. The anaesthetist followed the correct failed intubation procedure until a consultant arrived and intubated the trachea. No gastric contents were visible in the pharynx and the pulse oximeter readings were normal throughout the period of manual ventilation and intubation. A few minutes after delivery of the baby, the anaesthetists noted that increased airway pressures were required and that there was an expiratory wheeze. The arterial saturation decreased to 30% and bradycardia developed. The situation failed to respond to repositioning of the tube, or to repeated injections of aminophylline and hydrocortisone. Cardiac arrest occurred, external cardiac compression was started and adrenaline given. The tube cuff was then deflated and the tube moved down into the trachea and back again. This resulted in a great improvement in ventilation and the restoration of a normal cardiac rhythm. The patient was transferred to the Intensive Therapy Unit where fibre-optic bronchoscopy confirmed that the tube tended to enter the right main bronchus. The patient was weaned from the ventilator but had diffuse brain damage. After four weeks the patient ceased to tolerate the nasotracheal tube and it was agreed that a tracheostomy should be performed under general anaesthesia. This was initially uneventful, but inflation of the lungs through the tracheostomy tube proved impossible and the arterial saturation fell to 85%. Fibreoptic bronchoscopy revealed that the tube needed to be withdrawn 5cm in order to ensure that the tip did not enter the bronchus, but in this position there was too little tube in the trachea for safety. The tracheostomy tube was therefore removed and a tracheal tube inserted. At this point asystole developed which failed to respond to treatment.

Autopsy revealed that the immediate cause of death was widespread pulmonary embolization from pelvic and calf vein thromboses. The trachea was found to be 8cm long which, though short, was not unduly so for the patient's height (149cm), and there was no obvious anatomical abnormality to account for the difficulty with intubation. The tracheostomy incision was 5cm above the tracheal bifurcation. The cause of the difficulty with ventilation during the Caesarean section is still open to conjecture. No signs of aspiration were seen on laryngoscopy or on subsequent microscopical examination of the lungs and there were no signs of oedema on the postoperative X-ray. Later examination of the tracheal tube showed a weakness in part of the cuff which caused it to expand unevenly. This could have caused the cuff to herniate over the end of the tube or could have forced the open end of the tube against the wall of the trachea or medial wall of the right main bronchus. However, the fact that the ventilation improved rapidly after deflation of the cuff and repositioning of the tube, and that similar difficulties were encountered with the tracheostomy tube strongly suggests that the airway was obstructed by the passage of the tube into one bronchus. It should be standard practice *after every intubation* to listen to the breath sounds in each axilla (to ensure that the upper lobe bronchi are not obstructed) and to check the oxygen saturation continuously, for it may take several minutes for the oxygen saturation to decrease after a period of pre-oxygenation. If airway obstruction or wheezing develops in an intubated patient, the anaesthetist should first exclude a problem with the tube. Overinflation of the cuff or endobronchial intubation can be excluded by deflating the cuff and withdrawing the tube. If the problem persists the tube should be removed and a new tube substituted, care being taken to ensure that the top of the cuff lies 1–2cm below the vocal cords. This simple drill cures many instances of apparent "bronchospasm". However, it must be accepted that in this case there may have been some peculiar anatomical abnormality which was present in life and not apparent at autopsy, for similar complications occurred on each of the three occasions when the patient was anaesthetized by experienced consultants, who used recognized monitoring techniques, kept detailed records and apparently took the appropriate action after the complication developed.

Pulmonary oedema after spinal anaesthesia

An obese woman was admitted at 30 weeks gestation for drainage and marsupialisation of a recurrent Bartholin's abscess. The patient asked to be awake during the procedure and agreed to a spinal anaesthetic. She was premedicated with 15mg of papaveretum but was very nervous on arrival in the anaesthetic room, the pulse rate being 138–148/min (sinus rhythm), with a normal blood pressure and oxygen saturation. After a pre-load of 400ml of Hartmann's solution, 1ml of 0.5% heavy bupivacaine was injected in the sitting position with repeated aspiration of CSF to check that the needle was still in situ. After one minute the patient noticed some weakness of her legs. She was then placed in the supine position with the head resting on two pillows and the table tilted laterally. Six minutes after injection of the drug the blood pressure was recorded as 102/49mm Hg, with a pulse rate of 159bpm, and two minutes later it had fallen to 75/28mm Hg. The hypotension was treated initially by infusing a further 600ml of Hartmann's solution and giving two 15mg doses of ephedrine IV. These were followed by 600ml of synthetic colloid solution. Shortly after giving the ephedrine the pulse rate fell to 40–50/min with occasional ectopic beats for about 30 seconds. Oxygen was administered and followed by three doses of 0.6mg of atropine. Since the hypotension persisted, 1ml of 1:1,000 adrenaline was given IV. This produced a short period of bigemini, but ten minutes after the spinal the blood pressure was 135/86mm Hg and pulse rate 104. Since the patient had by now received 1000ml of Hartmann's solution and 600ml of colloid, the infusion was stopped. Approximately 20 minutes after the spinal injection the patient started to cough up pink, frothy sputum, and had a respiratory rate of 30/min, a blood pressure of 90/24mm Hg and pulse rate of 164/min, whilst the pulse oximeter showed an oxygen saturation of 80%. A total of 60mg of frusemide was given over the next 10 minutes and the patient was then given etomidate and suxamethonium to permit tracheal intubation and manual ventilation of the lungs. The abscess was drained and the patient transferred to the Intensive Therapy Unit. By the third postoperative day it had become apparent that she had developed severe ARDS and it was decided that a Caesarean section should be performed to decrease her oxygen requirement. Subsequently, renal failure and disseminated intravascular coagulation developed and continuous inotropic support was required. Death occurred 11 days after the spinal anaesthetic. There was no evidence of amniotic fluid embolism or any cardiac abnormality at autopsy.

It is difficult to differentiate sinus tachycardia from a tachyarrhythmia when the heart rate is in the range of 140–150bpm and the ECG is being displayed on a monitor screen. The sudden bradycardia after the fluid load and ephedrine suggests that the high heart rate was due to a tachyarrhythmia and it is unlikely that a cause for this would be apparent at autopsy. The dose of heavy bupivacaine used would not normally result in hypotension. This suggests that the hypotension was due to aortocaval compression resulting from the supine position, for a small degree of lateral tilt may not prevent this complication. In the presence of a tachycardia the combination of a fluid load and increase in afterload produced by the large doses of ephedrine and adrenaline could have precipitated severe pulmonary oedema, with the later development of ARDS.

Inadequate postoperative care

A very obese woman, who smoked 20 cigarettes a day, had chronic hypertension which was well controlled by atenolol. On admission the haemoglobin was 10.5g/dl, the blood pressure 180/90mm Hg and the patient was dyspnoeic at rest. She received a syntocinon infusion but had a prolonged first stage and was given epidural analgesia by request. Eight hours later it was decided that she should be delivered by Caesarean section. An experienced Registrar was called and asked to give a general anaesthetic since the patient refused to have the operation under epidural, even though this was working satisfactorily. General anaesthesia was uneventful, a dose of 20mg of papaveretum having been given intravenously after delivery of the baby. About 15 minutes after the patient had been extubated the midwife noted that she was cyanosed with laboured breathing, that the blood pressure was 70/30mm Hg, and the pulse rate 110bpm. The anaesthetist was called, gave an intravenous dose of naloxone and left. Twenty minutes later cardiac arrest occurred. The heart was restarted and the patient transferred to the Intensive Therapy Unit where she died five days later without recovering consciousness.

The anaesthetist failed to appreciate that the patient had been treated with atenolol, and that this, together with a residual epidural blockade, might lead to cardiovascular instability. The respiratory distress and hypotension could have been due to partial respiratory paralysis from continued action of the muscle relaxant or to undetected aspiration of gastric contents. However, the anaesthetist made no attempt to determine whether the respiratory distress was due to a central or peripheral cause by the use of a nerve stimulator. It seems likely that the problem had a cardiac origin. The autopsy revealed that the heart was enlarged, the coronary arteries were 30% occluded and there was fibrosis in the left ventricular myocardium, with vegetations on the mitral valve. It is probable that the combination of hypotension, anaemia and inadequate ventilation caused myocardial ischaemia which precipitated the cardiac arrest.

Possible aspiration of gastric contents

This woman was obese and smoked over 30 cigarettes per day. She had required a Caesarean section for her first child because of fetal distress and failure to progress, but her second pregnancy had resulted in a normal delivery. The third pregnancy proceeded normally until 34 weeks gestation when she was found to be anaemic. On the assumption that this was due to iron deficiency she was prescribed iron. However, the anaemia was macrocytic. She was admitted at 39 weeks with indigestion and vomiting and treated with ranitidine 150mg bd for three days. Labour was then induced but the head failed to engage and fetal tachycardia developed, so it was decided that she should have a Caesarean section under general anaesthesia. She had received ranitidine 50mg and pethidine 100mg IM two hours before operation, together with 800ml of crystalloid solution. The haemoglobin was 7.8g/dl. The anaesthetist, who was very experienced, was aware that the intubation had proved difficult at the last operation and noted that the patient had a short neck and receding chin. The patient was given 30ml of sodium citrate orally, placed supine with a left lateral tilt, and pre-oxygenated. Anaesthesia was then induced whilst cricoid pressure was applied. The larynx could not be visualised with a short blade but by substituting a long blade the anaesthetist was able to visualise the arytenoid cartilages and to intubate the trachea with the aid of a curved stilette. The patient did not become cyanosed and no gastric contents were observed in the pharynx. Anaesthesia was uneventful. One unit of packed cells was given during the first 20 minutes of the operation, a second unit during the next hour and a third unit during the next four hours. Blood loss was estimated to be 400ml. At the end of the operation ventilation was inadequate and two doses of atropine and neostigmine were given, though neuromuscular function was not tested with a nerve stimulator. Ventilation was assisted for the next 15 minutes and the tube was then removed with the patient in the supine position. It was noted that there were profuse pharyngeal secretions which were removed by a nasopharyngeal suction catheter. The patient was transferred to the recovery area and given 20mg of papaveretum and 12.5mg of prochlorperazine. Two hours after the end of the operation, when the patient was transferrred to the postnatal ward, the midwife noted that she was drowsy, and that she was "chesty" and wanted to cough. The blood pressure was 90/50mm Hg, the pulse rate 94bpm and the temperature 37.4°C. Four hours later the blood pressure was found to be 100/40mm Hg, the pulse rate 120bpm and the respiration rate 50/min. The midwife called the obstetric SHO who noted that the patient was restless and cyanosed. Blood-gas analysis showed that the arterial PO_2 was 5.8 kPa whilst breathing approximately 40% oxygen. Treatment with frusemide, hydrocortisone, antibiotics and nebulized salbutamol was started and the patient transferred to a medical ward for approximately five hours. Twelve hours after the end of the operation she was transferred to an Intensive Therapy Unit where she died ten days later from ARDS.

A number of factors could have affected the outcome in this case. A lack of communication between members of the obstetric team resulted in the patient being presented for operation with a haemoglobin of 7.8g/dl. The anaesthetist stated that no gastric contents were seen in the pharynx during intubation, but this manoeuvre proved difficult and the cords were not visualised. Gastric contents could have been aspirated at that time or after extubation in the supine position when "profuse secretions" had to be removed by blind nasopharyngeal suction. The anaesthetist did not empty the stomach during the operation. If this had been done, it would have reduced the risk of postoperative aspiration. The patient received 40mg of atracurium for muscle relaxation during the procedure. Since atracurium is normally destroyed by Hofmann degradation, it would have been expected that the action of the drug would have worn off by the end of the operation. However, the anaesthetist recorded that the patient was not breathing adequately and that two doses of atropine and neostigmine had to be given, though neuromuscular function was not tested by the use of a nerve stimulator. The fact that manual assistance to ventilation had to be provided for a further 15 minutes suggests that pulmonary oedema secondary to aspiration or fluid overload was already present. A CVP line should have been inserted to monitor the transfusion whilst the use of a pulse oximeter during and after operation would have revealed any defect in oxygen transfer and have led to earlier recognition of the pulmonary oedema. The postoperative care of this patient was considered to be substandard, for it was not until the day staff came on duty that a physician was called to see her. There was then a further delay of six hours before she was transferred to an Intensive Therapy Unit. The failure to respond to diuretics, the clinical course in the ITU and the autopsy findings all support the diagnosis of ARDS.

Late death

Aspiration of gastric contents

This patient died 45 days after the anaesthetic and has been counted as a *Late* death. She had a prolonged second stage with transverse arrest of the fetal head. Two 100mg doses of pethidine were given during labour. Since she had refused epidural analgesia, it was agreed that a trial of forceps should be undertaken under general anaesthesia. Metoclopramide 10mg and ranitidine 50mg were given intramuscularly and 10ml of of a proprietary antacid given orally. Anaesthesia was induced 20 minutes later with thiopentone and suxamethonium, cricoid pressure being applied by a trained assistant. The patient regurgitated a large quantity of gastric contents and laryngoscopy revealed that some had entered the trachea. Intubation was accomplished easily and the trachea aspirated, but the inflation pressure remained high despite the intravenous administration of aminophylline and methylprednisolone. The patient was transferred to the ITU but died from a suppurative bronchopneumonia and renal failure.

The anaesthetic was given by an experienced Registrar who was assisted by a trained operating department assistant. It is known that opioid drugs decrease gastric motility, and that metoclopramide has little effect on gastric emptying after they have been administered. Ranitidine decreases gastric acid secretion but this will have little effect on gastric pH if emptying is delayed. Since cricoid pressure prevents the regurgitation of gastric contents, even when the intragastric pressure is as high as 100cm of water, it must be concluded that the cricoid pressure was applied incorrectly or too late.

Deaths to which anaesthesia contributed

There were ten deaths in which it was considered that anaesthesia contributed to death. These have been counted in other chapters of this report, and are summarized in Table 9.3. In two patients the death was associated with haemorrhage and in two others there was pre-existing respiratory disease. The remaining six deaths were associated with substandard postoperative care.

Haemorrhage due to placenta percreta

The patient was admitted for elective Caesarean section because of a major degree of placenta praevia and a breech presentation. She had previously required an elective Caesarean section for breech presentation and pelvic disproportion. The patient asked the consultant anaesthetist to give an epidural anaesthetic. A 16 gauge venous cannula was inserted and 500ml of synthetic colloid and 1 litre of Hartmann's solution was administered over the ensuing 30 minutes. Satisfactory analgesia to T5 was produced by a total of 18ml of 0.5% bupivacaine. The placenta was abnormally adherent to the lower segment uterine wall and the registrar grade obstetrician, who attempted to remove it piecemeal, was unable to control the sudden profuse blood loss. Although the operation was taken over by a consultant obstetrician and a total of 26 units of blood, 6 units of human albumin, 4 units of fresh frozen plasma and 1 litre of synthetic colloid were administered over the next three hours, the patient succumbed.

Table 9.3 *Procedures requiring anaesthesia and causes of death in ten patients in whom anaesthesia contributed to death (ie excluding deaths directly due to anaesthesia)*

Obstetric procedure	Cause of death	Counted in Chapter
Emergency unplanned CS	Haemorrhage:placenta accreta	3
Laparotomy for ectopic pregnancy	ARDS (haemorrhage)	6
Surgical termination of pregnancy	Asthma	6
Emergency unplanned CS for fetal distress	Bronchopneumonia, renal failure, ? aspiration	12
Emergency planned CS for placental abruption	ARDS (?aspiration)	3
Emergency planned CS for fetal distress	Haemorrhage, epidural anaesthesia	3
Emergency unplanned CS for eclampsia	ARDS (?aspiration)	2
Laparotomy for ectopic pregnancy	ARDS (?aspiration)	6
Laparotomy for tubal pregnancy	Hypoxia, ?pulmonary oedema	6
Elective CS for pre-eclampsia	Hypoxia, ?airway obstruction	2

(For Caesarean section (CS) classification see Chapter 13).

The choice of epidural anaesthesia for such a patient is controversial as there is a high risk of severe haemorrhage. The normal cardiovascular responses may be impaired by the sympathetic blockade and surgical conditions may not be ideal in the conscious patient. Larger intravenous cannulae should have been used and a CVP line inserted for monitoring the transfusion. Caesarean section in a patient with a placenta praevia and a history of a previous section should only be undertaken by a very experienced obstetrician and anaesthetist.

Ectopic pregnancy: haemorrhagic hypotension and ARDS

This patient was admitted in a shocked state with an ectopic pregnancy. The blood pressure was unrecordable for the first 20 minutes of anaesthesia and blood loss was estimated as 60–80% of the blood volume. The patient had been transfused with one litre of synthetic colloid before induction and received a further two litres of colloid and four units of fresh frozen plasma before the fallopian tube was clamped. A CVP line was inserted at the end of the operation but shortly afterwards the patient developed hypotension and pulmonary oedema and had a cardiac arrest. After resuscitation a second laparotomy was performed to control continued bleeding and the patient transferred to an ITU, having received 16 units of blood, four units of fresh frozen plasma and three to four litres of colloid. At this time the CVP was 26cm H_2O. The pulmonary oedema cleared but ARDS developed and the patient died nine days later.

It is not clear when the consultant anaesthetist was called, but he did not arrive until after the cardiac arrest, so the anaesthetic was conducted by a registrar supported by an SHO. Although two units of O-negative blood were available in theatre before induction, and four units of the patient's group became available shortly afterwards, blood was not given until 30 minutes after induction when the cross-match had been confirmed. The replacement of red cells should not have been delayed until the cross-match was confirmed, for the excessive transfusion of colloids would have resulted in gross anaemia which would have compromised cardiac function and contributed to the occurrence of pulmonary oedema and cardiac arrest. This is a situation in which the clinical experience of a consultant anaesthetist could have contributed to the survival of the patient.

There were two deaths in which anaesthesia could have produced an exacerbation of pre-existing respiratory disease.

Bronchospasm during anaesthesia

A young woman, who presented for surgical termination of pregnancy at six weeks gestation, told both the gynaecologist and the general practitioner anaesthetist that she was asthmatic and required a salbutamol inhaler three to four times a day. She was admitted to the clinic on the morning of operation, premedicated with 5mg of diazepam and asked to take two puffs of salbutamol just before coming to theatre. Anaesthesia was induced with methohexitone 150mg and maintained with nitrous oxide-oxygen, 1ml of syntometrine being given during the procedure. The patient sneezed on being placed in the lithotomy position but breathed normally until the legs were taken down, when she developed difficulty in breathing and became cyanosed. She was given hydrocortisone 100mg and salbutamol 0.5mg intravenously. A tracheal tube was passed but manual ventilation with oxygen proved impossible because of severe bronchospasm. There was no response to a further dose of salbutamol and to two 1ml doses of 1/1000 adrenaline. Cardiac arrest occurred and the heart could not be defibrillated.

The patient had concealed the fact that she had suffered from very severe attacks of asthma, was being treated with inhaled steroids and had required inpatient treatment for asthma on a number of occasions. If the seriousness of her condition had been appreciated she would not have been treated in a private clinic. The cause of the acute bronchospasm is not clear. The fact that the patient "sneezed" on being placed in the lithotomy position suggests that she was very lightly anaesthetized and it is possible that she may have aspirated oral secretions or gastric contents. There was no record of any form of monitoring being used. The use of a pulse oximeter might have provided an earlier warning of arterial desaturation so that treatment could have been initiated earlier.

Bronchopneumonia with posssible gastric aspiration

> The patient had suffered a *Haemophilus influenzae* chest infection during her last pregnancy and in this pregnancy was admitted to hospital at 37 weeks gestation with a chest infection which was treated with erythromycin. Two days later she required a Caesarean section for fetal distress. The anaesthetic was carried out by an experienced registrar but he was unable to intubate the trachea. Whilst the anaesthetist was ventilating the patient by facemask the obstetrician found that the cervix was fully dilated and so delivered the infant *per vaginam* with forceps. Following delivery the trachea was intubated by a more senior anaesthetist. Although no gastric contents were seen in the pharynx, there was blood-stained fluid in the trachea. At the end of the operation the arterial PO_2 was low and there were bilateral infiltrations in the lung fields, so the patient was transferred to the ITU where she died six days later.

The patient had received antibiotics for two days before operation and was apparently recovering from the chest infection, but the chest X-ray taken shortly after operation showed bilateral infiltrates and the patient was severely hypoxic at this time. Although the autopsy report stated that this patient died from bronchopneumonia and renal failure and that there were no signs of ARDS, it is not possible to exclude possible aspiration as a result of the failed intubation.

In the remaining six cases it was considered that substandard postoperative care contributed to the patient's death.

Antepartum haemorrhage, possible aspiration , ARDS

> A young woman required a Caesarean section for an antepartum haemorrhage. She had been given 150mg of ranitidine orally six hours previously. There were no problems with the general anaesthetic but the patient vomited once in the lateral position when conscious in the recovery area. There was a delay in obtaining cross-matched blood and the estimated 1.5–2 litres blood loss was replaced with colloid during the operation, two units of blood being given during the postoperative period. Papaveretum 15mg was given intramuscularly one hour after the end of the anaesthetic and another 20mg given 80 minutes later. After two hours a further 30 mg was given. One hour later the patient was found to

be cyanosed and dyspnoeic. 40mg of frusemide was given IV and the patient transferred to the ITU where she died 10 days later from ARDS.

The clinical course was compatible with an aspiration of gastric contents but there was no recorded difficulty during the anaesthetic and it is unlikely that the patient would have aspirated when she vomited soon after regaining consciousness in the recovery ward. However, she subsequently received a total of 65mg of papaveretum within a period of four hours. It is possible that the failure to achieve adequate analgesia with the initial doses of papaveretum was due to impaired absorption in a hypovolaemic patient. A subsequent improvement in haemodynamic status might then have resulted in the absorption of all the papaveretum. This could have caused a diminished level of consciousness and aspiration of gastric contents. The problem could have been avoided by administering the opioid by the intravenous route during the period of hypovolaemia. There was a singular lack of postoperative observations and it is considered that the postoperative monitoring and supervision were substandard.

Postpartum haemorrhage and epidural anaesthesia

> This lady required an emergency Caesarean section for fetal distress. She had received epidural analgesia for pain relief three hours before and this was extended to T6/7 by injection of two 10ml doses of 0.5% bupivacaine. Blood loss was minimal and the patient was conscious and pain free on transfer to the recovery area. On two occasions during the next hour the midwife recorded that clear urine was draining from the catheter and that blood pressure, pulse rate and wound drainage were normal. Forty minutes later the patient was found to be unrousable. Resuscitation was attempted without success.

Autopsy showed extensive haemorrhage into parametrial tissues and some 500ml of blood in the right paracolic gutter. Death was attributed to the effects of haemorrhage in the presence of continuing epidural blockade. It is possible that the failure to recognise the complication was due to the fact that the signs of intra-abdominal haemorrhage may be modified by the presence of continuing sympathetic and sensory blockade, but the paucity of postoperative observations suggests that postoperative care was inadequate. There was a delay in initiating resuscitation because the maternity unit was situated some distance from the general hospital, but this is unlikely to have affected the outcome because of the initial delay in recognising the arrest.

Eclampsia, possible aspiration, ARDS

> A young primiparous woman had been admitted to hospital at 35 weeks gestation with diarrhoea and vomiting, thought to be due to gastroenteritis. Shortly after admission she had an eclamptic fit and it was decided to perform an immediate Caesarean section.

The patient was given diazepam and chlormethiazole and was barely conscious on arrival in theatre. She received an uneventful general anaesthetic, but there is no record of the administration of an H_2 blocking drug, or of the stomach being emptied during anaesthesia. The postoperative records are scanty but it appears that she received 3.5 litres of fluid, of which 2 litres were colloid, during the first 12 hours, though the CVP line was apparently not working. The patient died ten days later from ARDS.

No precautions were taken to minimise the risk of postoperative aspiration, the anaesthetic record is missing and the junior anaesthetist does not appear to have discussed the case with a senior colleague. Post-operative care and the control of fluid balance appeared to be grossly deficient. It is possible that the ARDS resulted from aspiration during the eclamptic fit or in the postoperative period.

Ectopic pregnancy, possible aspiration

An obese, anxious woman presented with an ectopic pregnancy of eight weeks gestation. Resuscitation, anaesthesia and surgery were uneventful and fluid balance was monitored by an internal jugular line. She required a total of 40mg of papaveretum in the first six hours after operation, but was then transferred to patient-controlled analgesia with 4mg bolus doses of morphine, a 10 minute lockout period and a background infusion of 1mg/hour. Seven hours later the nurse noted that the breathing was laboured; three hours after this the patient was noted to be stuporose and foaming at the mouth. During this ten hour period she had received a total of 73mg of morphine. Investigations revealed a PO_2 of 3.6kPa, PCO_2 of 5.9kPa and a WBC of 36,400. A blood culture taken at this time grew gram negative bacilli, but these could not be identified. Naloxone and oxygen were administered and the patient transferred to an ITU, but the chest condition worsened and she died 14 days later with ARDS.

Postoperatively the patient had paralytic ileus, abdominal distension, and signs of developing sepsis, but no attempt was made to empty the stomach and oxygen administration was discontinued ten hours after the end of the operation. The patient was anxious and distressed by the loss of the pregnancy and patient-controlled analgesia was a logical choice for pain relief. However, the use of a background infusion, together with large bolus doses, increases the risks of respiratory depression. In the absence of oxygen therapy, the resulting hypoxia, augmented by obesity and abdominal distension, together with developing sepsis, may have depressed the level of consciousness and so contributed to the aspiration of gastric contents which was confirmed at autopsy.

Ectopic pregnancy , possible fluid overload

This woman was a heavy smoker who was operated on for a tubal pregnancy. The Hb was 7.9g/dl before operation and four units of blood and one litre of colloid were given during the operation. The anaesthetic was uneventful and the patient was awake on transfer to a single room where she was subsequently nursed. Eighteen hours later she had a cardiac arrest. There was conflicting evidence concerning fluid balance during this period, but it seems probable that input exceeded output by 3.5 litres. She had also received three doses of 20mg of papaveretum for pain relief, the last dose being given within two hours of the arrest.

The cardiac arrest could have been caused by pulmonary oedema or by hypoxia resulting from excessive doses of opioid drug (she weighed 49kg), but its occurrence emphasises the dangers of nursing patients in isolated surroundings after operation. The continuous monitoring of arterial saturation by pulse oximeter would have given warning of hypoxia due to respiratory depression or pulmonary oedema.

Pre-eclampsia, possible airway obstruction

A young primigravida, who suffered from mild asthma, developed pre-eclampsia and was admitted to hospital at 34 weeks gestation. One week later she developed vomiting, headache, visual disturbances and epigastric pain with a blood pressure of 140/105mm Hg and oedema, but only a trace of protein in the urine. She was treated with diazepam and arrangements made for a Caesarean section. There had been great difficulties with tracheal intubation for a laparoscopy some two years previously, so the section was performed under a spinal anaesthetic with 3ml of 0.5% heavy bupivacaine and sedation with midazolam 5mg IV. After operation the patient was alert and appeared to be in a stable circulatory state with a good urinary output and minimal proteinuria, so she was transferred to the postnatal ward. Two hours after delivery she was given 20mg of papaveretum for pain relief and four hours later she received another 20mg plus 10mg of diazepam. A further 10mg of papaveretum was given two hours later for continuing headache and restlessness. Two hours after this she was found to have had a cardiac arrest which did not respond to resuscitative measures.

This patient should have been monitored in a high dependency area for at least 24 hours to ensure that the pre-eclampsia was resolving. It was observed that she snored heavily when asleep though she had no clinical history of sleep apnoea. Pulse oximetry studies have now revealed that patients with episodes of airway obstruction during sleep may develop marked arterial desaturation, together with acute increases of pulse rate and blood pressure during the period of obstruction, and that these changes are much greater after the administration of sedative and analgesic drugs. The only trained midwife on the ward had to leave temporarily to help in another ward at the presumed time of the death, but even if she had been present, she might not have detected this problem in a darkened ward. The requirement for opioid drugs could have been reduced by the use of epidural analgesia postoperatively, whilst monitoring by pulse oximeter might have revealed episodes of arterial desaturation. It is likely that this tragedy could have been avoided if the patient's care had been supervised by senior medical staff and she had been nursed in a properly equipped and staffed recovery or high-dependency area.

Comment

A comparison of the deaths associated with anaesthesia in the present triennium with those listed in the last report is not considered justifiable because the total number of deaths is small and, in some cases, the information made available to the assessors was very limited. Nevertheless, the decrease in deaths directly due to anaesthesia observed in the last triennium appears to have been maintained. It is notable that there were no deaths due to unrecognised oesophageal intubation. It seems unlikely that this improvement can be attributed to the introduction of CO_2 monitors since the Association of Anaesthetists' publication "Recommendations for standard of monitoring during anaesthesia and recovery" was not published until 1988, and there was an inevitable delay of several years before the recommendations could be fully implemented. Nevertheless, there is now strong evidence that the presence of CO_2 in the expired gas provides the only certain way of ensuring that the tube is in the trachea.

It is recommended that a CO_2 analyser should be provided in all locations where a general anaesthetic is administered.

In this triennium there was one death due directly to a tracheal tube problem and one to obvious aspiration of gastric contents. In a number of other cases aspiration during anaesthesia or the postoperative period could have contributed to death, but when death is delayed for a week or more after the primary event it is difficult to obtain evidence of aspiration at autopsy. Whilst there is general agreement that H_2 blocking drugs should be administered prophylactically to all women in labour who are likely to require a regional or general anaesthetic, there is no consensus concerning their use in those expected to have a normal labour. The prophylactic administration of H_2 blocking drugs and a non-particulate antacid, such as sodium citrate, can reduce the risk of lung damage due to inhalation of gastric contents, but the effectiveness of these drugs is reduced if gastric emptying has been delayed by a prolonged labour or the administration of opioid drugs. These factors, and the unpredictable need for a general anaesthetic for such emergencies as a prolapsed cord, provide support for the view that H_2 blockers should be considered for all women in labour. Others consider that cost considerations and the possibility of side effects demands a more conservative approach. However, the fact that ARDS was the ultimate cause of death in 18.5% of the *Direct* and *Indirect* deaths in this triennium, and that 41% of these also had a hypertensive disorder of pregnancy, suggests that all patients with pre-eclampsia should receive an H_2 blocking drug when they go into labour. There may also still be a case for reconsidering the role of pre-operative gastric aspiration in women who have had a prolonged labour or inadequate pre-operative preparation. Since there is evidence that the prophylactic administration of H_2 blocking drugs may not always result in the desired increase in pH, it should be routine practice to empty the stomach through an oral gastric tube during operation to reduce the risk of postoperative aspiration. It would also be worth considering measurement of the pH of the aspirate with indicator paper and the administration of further sodium citrate if the pH is less than 2.5.

H_2 receptor blocking drugs should be administered to all patients who may require anaesthesia, and to patients with pre-eclampsia. A non-particulate antacid should also be given before induction of general anaesthesia. In patients in whom delayed gastric emptying is suspected, pre-operative emptying of the stomach should be considered. The stomach should be routinely emptied before extubation to minimise the risks of postoperative aspiration.

The treatment of haemorrhage is still a matter of some concern. This is due partly to difficulties in assessing the extent of the blood loss, particularly when the haemorrhage occurs over an extended period, and partly to the fact that the emergency is usually dealt with by relatively inexperienced junior staff who tend to underestimate blood loss, and to assume that the blood volume is not seriously depleted if the blood pressure is normal.

It should be standard practice to insert large bore IV cannulae and a CVP line, and to call for more senior obstetric and anaesthetic assistance as soon as severe blood loss is observed or suspected. Guidelines such as those given in the annexe to Chapter 3, concerning the provision of blood and blood products for obstetric emergencies, and involvement of a haematologist should be implemented in every unit.

A number of deaths were due to a lack of adequate postoperative care. There are still a number of obstetric units where high dependency care facilities are inadequate and where the responsibility for medical and nursing care is not clearly defined.

Midwifery staff deputed to look after postoperative patients should be specifically trained in monitoring, the care of the airway and resuscitative procedures and should be supervised by a defined anaesthetist at all times.

It is helpful to provide a written check list to ensure that all new staff are fully aware of departmental policies and procedures, and all staff should receive regular refresher courses to ensure that they perform with optimal efficiency.

Monitoring by pulse oximeter throughout anaesthesia and the early postoperative period should be routine. Pulse oximetry should be continued for longer periods whenever the patient's condition gives ground for concern. In some circumstances pulse oximetry may need to be continued through the first or second postoperative nights, for pulmonary complications often produce maximal arterial desaturation at this time.

Most anaesthetic departments now provide a postoperative pain relief service and this should be extended to cover postoperative maternity patients.

This Report has highlighted the relatively high incidence of ARDS in deaths associated with pregnancy (see Annexe to this chapter). In a number of these cases ARDS was associated with well known predisposing factors such as the aspiration of gastric contents, pneumonia, sepsis and haemorrhagic shock, but in other cases there was no clear cause. Since many of the patients also had a history of a hypertensive disorder of pregnancy it would seem that this association needs further investigation.

Table 9.4 *Predisposing factors in 44 patients dying with the Adult Respiratory Distress Syndrome*

Predisposing factor	Number of patients
Haemorrhage or hypotension	12
Aspiration	10
Sepsis	6
Pneumonia	11
Miscellaneous	5

Great strides have been made in the provision of dedicated consultant sessions for obstetric anaesthesia during the past decade, but the direct supervision and training of junior staff by consultants is still inadequate in a number of hospitals.

The provision of adequate consultant supervision is particularly difficult in the smaller hospitals and in those with separate maternity units and every effort should be made to bring maternity services onto the main hospital site.

Annexe to Chapter 9

Adult Respiratory Distress Syndrome (ARDS)

Summary

Forty four of the 238 *Direct* and *Indirect* deaths in the present triennium were associated with the development of the Adult Respiratory Distress Syndrome (ARDS). The presumed initiating factors for the ARDS were aspiration (10 patients), chest infection (11 patients), haemorrhage or hypotension (12 patients) and sepsis (6 patients). Three were due to hepatic failure complicating eclampsia and the remaining two to tracheal burns and cerebral haemorrrhage. Eighteen of the 44 patients (41%) had a hypertensive disorder of pregnancy.

The syndrome was first described in 1967[1] and the possible aetiology has been recently reviewed[2]. The most common clinical disorders associated with the development of ARDS are sepsis (30–40% of all cases) and aspiration of gastric contents (30–35%). About 25% of all cases have received multiple blood transfusions. ARDS also occurs in patients with pulmonary contusion, bone fractures, near-drowning, burns, cardiopulmonary bypass or drug overdose. Patients with staphylococcal or influenzal pneumonia often develop lung changes which are similar to ARDS.

In 80% of patients who develop ARDS the onset is within 24 hours of the initial insult. There is evidence that lung changes occur within six hours of the development of sepsis and that the onset may be even earlier in patients who aspirate gastric contents. The patient develops increasing respiratory distress, with severe hypoxaemia due to right-to-left intrapulmonary shunting, and widespread infiltrates are seen on the chest X-ray. Although the hypoxaemia may be reduced by the administration of oxygen and continuous positive pressure breathing, mechanical assistance to ventilation is usually required. High airway pressures are needed to maintain adequate ventilation in the presence of a greatly reduced lung compliance and positive end-expiratory pressure (PEEP) is usually applied to increase lung volume, and so reduce the alveolar collapse. The resulting high inflation pressures often result in barotrauma. A number of other ventilatory modes may be used to minimise inflation pressures, but neither these, nor the various methods of extracorporeal lung support, have been shown to affect the mortality. Infection commonly complicates treatment and death usually results from multi-organ failure.

The initial changes in the lung are due to increased permeability of the pulmonary capillaries which results in interstitial and alveolar oedema and alveolar collapse. It has been suggested that the increased permeability is due to damage to the pulmonary endothelium associated with the presence of large numbers of inflammatory cells, mainly neutrophils, which are found in the the air spaces and interstitium of the lung at this time. There is also evidence that there may be destruction of the alveolar epithelium. This is important because it may lower the threshold for alveolar flooding and so further impair gas exchange. Five to ten days after the initial insult there is a pronounced increase in collagen and fibroblast formation in the interstitium of the lung with an increase in Type II cells lining the alveoli. After two weeks there is considerable lung destruction with areas of emphysema, pulmonary vascular obliteration and fibrosis. During this phase oxygenation usually improves but there is still a large physiological dead space so that minute volumes of 15–20 litres are required to maintain normal carbon dioxide levels. Although the lung has a liver-like appearance at autopsy and the normal lung architecture often appears to have been almost completely destroyed, the primary cause of death is usually multiple organ failure. Whether this is related to the original insult or to the effects of treatment is not known.

The reported mortality rate in patients with ARDS varies widely because of lack of uniformity in diagnostic criteria, differences in aetiology and variations in treatment. For example, the mortality rate in patients with sepsis appears to be approximately 90%, whilst that associated with fat embolism is about 10%. It has been suggested that the mortality in patients who have aspirated gastric contents may be predicted from blood-gas measurements. For example, Bynum and Pierce[3] measured the blood-gases of 44 patients within 1 hour of aspiration and calculated the ratio of measured arterial oxygen tension to calculated alveolar oxygen tension. If the ratio was 0.5 or less the mortality rate was 48%: if greater than 0.5 it was 14%. Whether these results would appply to pregnant patients is not known.

There is little information on the incidence of ARDS in obstetric patients. In one University obstetric unit with 21,983 deliveries over a five-year period there were 23 pregnancy-related admissions to an Intensive Therapy Unit. The most frequent cause of admission was a hypertensive disorder of pregnancy and the majority of these cases required admission for less than two days. Three patients were diagnosed as having ARDS and two of these died[4]. During the ensuing four year period (1989–92) in the same unit there were only ten pregnancy-related ITU admissions associated with 19,685 deliveries, seven of these patients having a hypertensive disorder of pregnancy. In this period there were no patients with ARDS and all of the patients survived[5].

In the 44 cases of ARDS identified in this triennium, and listed in Table 9.4, there were three in which there was strong evidence of aspiration of gastric contents, and seven cases where aspiration was presumed because of the rapid onset of respiratory failure after a situation where aspiration could have occurred. Six of these ten cases were associated with eclampsia. Eleven patients had pneumonia which progressed to ARDS whilst 12 patients had suffered severe hypotension or haemorrhage. The observation that 18 out of the 44 patients with ARDS (41%) had a hypertensive disorder of pregnancy, suggests that this association requires further study. It is known that patients with pre-eclampsia are at increased risk of developing pulmonary oedema, but this usually resolves with suitable treatment in the postpartum period. Since cardiogenic oedema does not usually result in ARDS, and since patients with epileptiform fits rarely develop ARDS unless aspiration occurs, it would seem that the development of ARDS in pregnant patients must be associated with some pregnancy or pre-eclamptic induced changes in the lung which predispose to the development of this condition. Whether such changes could lead to the development of ARDS when aspiration has not occurred is unknown. In the absence of such information it is recommended that particular attention should be paid to the prevention of aspiration in this group of patients by the prophylactic administration of H_2 blocking drugs before and after operation, by emptying the stomach during anaesthesia and by the use of high dependency care for at least 24 hours after delivery.

References

1. Ashbaugh DG, Bigelow DB, Petty TL, Levene BE. Acute Respiratory Distress in adults. *Lancet* 1967;**2**:319–323.
2. Wiener-Kronish JP, Gropper MA, Matthay MA. The adult respiratory distress syndrome: definition and prognosis, pathogenesis and treatment. *Br.J.Anaesth.* 1990;**65**:107–129.
3. Bynum LJ, Pierce AK. Pulmonary aspiration of gastric contents. *Amer. Rev. Resp. Dis.* 1976;**114**:1129–1136.
4. Graham SG, Luxton MC. The requirement for intensive care support for the pregnant population. *Anaesthesia* 1989;**44**:581–584.
5. Luxton MC. Personal communication.

CHAPTER 10

Other Direct Deaths

Summary

Other *Direct* Deaths comprise those due to miscellaneous causes not dealt with in other chapters and also those where the cause was not conclusively determined.

There were 14 such deaths in this triennium. In nine the cause was clearly established and autopsies had been performed in eight. In the other five the cause was doubtful; in one of these an autopsy had not been done. There were three additional deaths; one, associated with a hypertensive disorder of pregnancy and acute fatty liver, is counted in Chapter 2; another from disseminated intravascular coagulation (DIC) following induction for missed abortion, is counted in Chapter 3; and the third from breast abscess and septicaemia occurred late and is counted in Chapter 15.

Liver Diseases

Liver abnormalities associated with hypertensive disorders of pregnancy are counted and discussed in Chapter 2. There were five other *Direct* deaths associated with acute fatty liver which are counted in this chapter. Although jaundice occurred in four of these it was not a prominent presenting feature in any. General malaise, nausea and vomiting were the commonest early symptoms. The management of all these patients was regarded as satisfactory.

> In a multipara with polyhydramnios the membranes ruptured spontaneously at 37 weeks gestation and labour ensued; soon afterwards she had a generalised convulsion. Emergency Caesarean section was performed on account of fetal distress. She developed signs of coagulation defect including severe postpartum haemorrhage. Cardiac failure supervened and did not respond to resuscitative measures and she died three and a half hours after delivery. Although the precise cause of death was not apparent at autopsy, the presence of acute fatty liver and DIC was confirmed.
>
> A parous woman complained of nausea and vomiting at 34 weeks gestation and was slightly jaundiced. Investigation disclosed early coagulation disorder and hepato-renal disfunction. A tentative diagnosis of acute fatty liver was made and she was deliv-

ered by Caesarean section. Her condition deteriorated and a liver transplant was performed seven days after delivery. Although this was technically successful she never regained consciousness and died two days later. The diagnosis of acute fatty liver was confirmed histologically.

A young parous woman was admitted at 35 weeks gestation with abdominal pain. Two days later she complained of nausea and vomiting and her serum bilirubin was elevated. She went into labour the same day and was delivered normally. Thereafter jaundice became evident and she rapidly went into renal and hepatic failure, became comatose and died 29 hours after delivery. Autopsy confirmed the diagnosis of acute fatty liver.

A multipara complained of dyspepsia at 34 weeks gestation. Next day she went into premature labour. Caesarean section was performed for fetal distress and jaundice was first noticed. Signs of hepatorenal failure rapidly developed and she was transferred to an Intensive Therapy Unit (ITU) ten hours after delivery. Adult Respiratory Distress Syndrome (ARDS) complicated the hepatorenal failure and despite appropriate expert therapy she died 34 hours after delivery.

A young primigravida at 36 weeks gestation was considered to have intrauterine fetal growth retardation. Labour was induced by amniotomy and abnormalities were detected in the fetal heart rate tracing. Caesarean section was therefore performed. Two days later she complained of feeling unwell with nausea and vomiting. She became jaundiced and liver function tests were abnormal; a diagnosis of acute fatty liver was made. Her condition deteriorated rapidly despite appropriate therapy. Cardiac arrest supervened and resuscitative efforts were unavailing. She died 52 hours after delivery.

The husband of one of these unfortunate patients had, not surprisingly, great difficulty in understanding how this calamity had befallen his wife, despite all the recent advances in medical and obstetric practice. At his request the records and the autopsy material were reviewed in another expert department and the findings confirmed. The patient's obstetrician received a detailed and very helpful letter from the Director of the Liver Unit concerned, who pointed out that, although the overall mortality from acute fatty liver of pregnancy has decreased, it still, despite recent advances, accounts for a number of maternal deaths each year and as its aetiology is not yet understood there is no way of preventing it at present. It is worth re-emphasising the value of having a second opinion, as experienced and as expert as possible, when attempting to comfort and reassure grieving relatives in such difficult and distressing cases.

Direct Deaths Due to Bacterial Infection

There were two such deaths, the causative organism being *Clostridium difficile* in one and beta haemolytic streptococcus in the other. A third death from septicaemia associated with a breast abscess is considered in Chapter 15 as the death occurred 51 days postpartum.

> A teenage primigravida was first seen at the antenatal clinic at 37 weeks gestation. She was subsequently delivered at term by Caesarean section because of an abnormal fetal heart rate tracing associated with a persistent occipito-posterior position and a prolonged first stage. The next day she was pyrexial and remained so despite antibiotic therapy. On the third day her abdomen was distended and tender, associated with diarrhoea. Sigmoidoscopy on the fourth day by a surgical registrar showed only faecal fluid in the bowel. On the fifth day a surgical consultant performed laparotomy. There was no evidence of peritonitis but the large gut was very hyperaemic and distended with fluid. The abdomen was closed and sigmoidoscopy repeated. There was now extensive sloughing and ulceration of the upper rectum and sigmoid colon. Rectal biopsy and stool for culture were taken and confirmed a diagnosis of pseudomembranous colitis due to *Clostridium difficile* infection. She was transferred to an ITU but failed to respond to therapy and died 11 days post-operatively.

Pseudomembranous colitis is caused by the toxin of *Clostridium difficile* which colonises the colon. Most cases develop after broad spectrum antibiotic therapy of which ampicillin, clindamycin and lincomycin are most frequently implicated. It is relevant that this patient received co-amoxiclav (Augmentin) which has a similar antibacterial spectrum to ampicillin.

> A young primigravida failed to attend the antenatal clinic from 30 weeks gestation. After 35 weeks she was seen by the community midwives on five occasions at home because of raised blood pressure. She was delivered at term by Caesarean section for severe pre-eclampsia, the cervix being unsuitable for induction of labour. She seemed normal when observed by a midwife 11 hours after delivery. Half an hour later she was found dead in bed. Autopsy unexpectedly revealed DIC and septicaemia with beta haemolytic streptococci.

Both these patients were socially deprived and their antenatal care was compromised by their poor attendance. Otherwise there was no reason to regard their management as substandard.

Deaths without satisfactory explanation

There were a total of nine such deaths in this triennium; five counted in this chapter, and the others in chapters 2 and 12. Of the five deaths where no adequate cause could be determined, two were antenatal and three postnatal. In four the management was considered to be satisfactory; autopsies had been performed in all of these. In the fifth the records were so incomplete as to preclude any accurate assessment; an autopsy had not been done here. Another death, where the cause was not entirely clear, was associated with a hypertensive disorder of pregnancy and is counted in Chapter 2. There were three other unexplained deaths which are counted in Chapter 12.

A young primigravida was found dead in bed at home at 34 weeks gestation, apparently having had a fit. During this pregnancy she had developed gestational diabetes but was otherwise normal when last seen at the antenatal clinic 20 days before her death. Autopsy failed to provide an explanation for this death, apparently the result of a fit, the cause of which was not determined. There was no evidence of pre-eclampsia or other pathology, and no history, before or during this pregnancy, of epilepsy. In these circumstances this death must be regarded as unexplained.

A young woman in the 32nd week of a normal pregnancy was found lying unconscious in her home. She was taken by ambulance to a casualty department where cardiac arrest and intra-uterine death were diagnosed. A diagnosis of intra-abdominal bleeding was made and successful resuscitation was followed by laparotomy. Severe generalised abdominal haemorrhage was discovered and splenectomy was performed on the assumption that the spleen was ruptured. When this was disproved, hysterectomy, with the fetus in utero, was carried out. Generalised uncontrollable bleeding, suggestive of DIC, continued unabated and the patient died in theatre four hours after admission. Autopsy confirmed DIC; the fetus was not macerated. Amniotic fluid embolism was considered as the likeliest cause of the DIC, but despite careful histological search, could not be demonstrated. The primary pathology must be regarded as undetermined.

A parous woman in her thirties was delivered at 35 weeks gestation by Caesarean section because of poorly controlled diabetes mellitus and previous Caesarean section. On the next day she was pyrexial and antibiotic therapy was begun. Bacteriology at this time proved negative and remained so. On the third post-operative day she became hypotensive and responded poorly to IV therapy. On the fourth day ascites was noted and paracentesis was performed, drawing off a litre of sterile fluid. Later that day she developed cardio-respiratory arrest, and despite attempts at resuscitation died shortly afterwards on the fourth post-operative day. Autopsy failed to reveal a convincing cause of death. Septicaemic toxaemia was suspected but all antemortem bacteriology was negative and postmortem blood culture — 48 hours after death - grew klebsiella only after prolonged incubation.

A teenage primigravida was first seen in the ante-natal clinic at 13 weeks gestation. Her haemoglobin was 10.9g/dl; it was not repeated thereafter. Her BP was normal throughout the pregnancy, but when admitted at term in early labour she was found to have severe pre-eclampsia, BP 150/110mg Hg, heavy proteinuria, oedema and headache. The hypertension responded to epidural bupivicaine and she was delivered by vacuum extraction. She lost 300-600 ml of blood postpartum. Next day she was pale and tired and complained of headache; she was now normotensive. Her haemoglobin on the second day was 5.6g/dl and she was transfused with one unit of packed cells and three units of blood, whereupon she developed signs of left ventricular failure. This improved after oxygen and intravenous frusemide. The next day she was found in the toilet unconscious and twitching. After transfer to the high dependency unit (HDU) she had two more convulsions and was moved to an ITU. Despite appropriate therapy she developed increasing evidence of ARDS. Eventually renal failure supervened and she died five weeks after delivery. Autopsy confirmed the presence of ARDS. The initial obstetric condition and the cause of the convulsions three and four days after delivery remained obscure.

Another teenage primigravida was admitted at 31 weeks gestation, possibly with abruptio placentae — the records are very inadequate. Labour was induced with prostaglandin pessaries and syntocinon infusion. During labour her BP rose to 230/170mm Hg; it was controlled with IV hypotensive drugs and she was delivered spontaneously of a stillborn male infant. Next day her condition deteriorated and she was transferred to an ITU where she died 11 days later; no autopsy was performed. The death certificate gives cardiac failure from septicaemia as the cause of death.

In view of the lack of essential evidence this death is classified as without satisfactory explanation.

Accidental Death due to Aortic Puncture

A young woman had recurrent severe hyperemesis from the third month of pregnancy. This required repeated intravenous therapy and, from the 27th week, total parenteral feeding through a CVP line. At the 33rd week the IV catheter had to be replaced. This was done, via the internal jugular vein, in the operating theatre by the anaesthetic registrar. Soon afterwards cardiac arrest occurred and efforts to resuscitate the patient failed. Postmortem Caesarean section was performed; the baby was stillborn. Autopsy indicated that the maternal death was caused by cardiac tamponade from a haemopericardium due to puncture of the ascending aorta by a needle inserted deeply into the internal jugular vein.

Death associated with Trophoblastic Disease

A young parous woman presented with vaginal bleeding in the 17th week of pregnancy. The uterus corresponded to 28 weeks in size and ultrasonic scan showed a hydatidiform mole. The patient refused admission but came into hospital that evening after a severe vaginal haemorrhage. Her haemoglobin was 5.3 g/dl and blood was transfused and the uterus evacuated by suction. She collapsed and chest X-ray showed diffuse mottling, suggestive of multiple microemboli; pulmonary aspirate contained trophoblastic cells. She was transferred to an ITU where despite appropriate treatment including chemotherapy with methotrexate and folic acid, she died two weeks later. Clinically there was evidence of a cerebro-vascular accident, possibly haemorrhage into a cerebral secondary choriocarcinoma; but in the rather unsatisfactory records there was no histological or biochemical evidence of this and no autopsy had been performed.

Comment

If the number of unsatisfactorily explained deaths is to be reduced in future, the responsible consultant obstetricians must endeavour to ensure that complete and accurate clinical records and autopsy reports are available for study. That this is still not the case is apparent.

CHAPTER 11

Cardiac Disease

Summary

There were 21 deaths associated with cardiac disease. Eighteen were *Indirect* and are counted in this chapter. A *Fortuitous* death is counted in Chapter 14 and two *Late* deaths are counted in Chapter 15.

Ten (56%) of the 18 patients were primigravidae, compared with 38% in the previous triennium, and four (22%) patients were aged under 25 compared with 38% in 1985–87.

Substandard care was considered to be present in 16 of the 18 cases (89%). This includes seven patients who refused to accept advice or treatment.

Congenital heart disease accounted for 9(50%) cardiac deaths. The proportion of deaths from congenital disease continues to increase.

There were 18 *Indirect* deaths associated with cardiac disease which are counted in this chapter. There was also a *Fortuitous* death due to acute viral myocarditis which is counted in Chapter 14. Two *Late* deaths, one due to coronary thrombosis and the other to acute cardiac failure, are counted in Chapter 15.

Nine deaths were due to complications of congenital heart disease and nine to aquired disease (Table 11.1). The diagnoses are listed in Table 11.2.

Congenital heart disease

Congenital heart disease accounted for 9(50%) cardiac deaths. The number of cases has remained fairly static but they have constituted an increasing proportion of deaths through the period of the Reports for England and Wales. In the first UK Report (1985–87) the proportion was 43%.

Substandard care

There was considered to be substandard care in eight of the nine cases of congenital disease. In three the patient had become pregnant in spite of professional advice to the contrary, had refused termination of pregnancy and/or had failed to comply with prescribed treatment. These were a woman with pulmonary hypertension who was awaiting a heart/lung transplant, one with Fallot's tetralogy and one with hypertrophic obstructive cardiomyopathy.

Table 11.1 *Number of maternal deaths from congenital and acquired cardiac diseases England and Wales during 1973–90 and United Kingdom*

	Congenital	Acquired Ischaemic	Acquired Other	Acquired Total	All Cases
England & Wales					
1973–75	4	N/A	N/A	14	18
1976–78	3	N/A	N/A	14	17
1979–81	4	6	6	12	16
1982–84	6	8	3	11	17
1985–87	10	6	3	9	19
1988–90	6	4	4	8	14
United Kingdom					
1985–87	10	9	4	13	23
1988–90	9	5	4	9	18

Table 11.2 *Maternal deaths due to cardiac diseases*

Congenital		9
Fallot's tetralogy	1	
Patent ductus arteriosus	1	
Transposition of great vessels	1	
Aortic stenosis	1	
Atrial septal defect	1	
Pulmonary hypertension	2	
Repaired atrial septal defect, endomyocardial fibroelastosis	1	
Hypertrophic obstructive cardiomyopathy	1	
Acquired		9
Ischaemic heart disease	4	
Mitral valve disease	2	
Dilated cardiomyopathy	2	
Familial ß hyperlipidaemia, atheroma	1	

The five cases in which there was substandard professional care are described below:

> A case of *primary pulmonary hypertension* was unrecognised even when the patient developed signs indicative of heart disease at 26 weeks gestation. She was delivered by Caesarean section and died five days later.

A woman with an unrecognised *atrial septal defect* received an over-load of fluid during induction of labour. She became breathless and cyanosed during labour and whilst she was being positioned for ventouse delivery she had a cardiac arrest and could not be resus-citated. The diagnosis of atrial septal defect was only made at autopsy.

A *patent ductus with right-left shunt* was not diagnosed antenatally in a woman who had a history of cardiological supervision in childhood and clubbing of her fingers. She had an antepartum haemorrhage and was delivered by Caesarean section. This was followed by a secondary postpartum haemorrhage and she died four days post partum.

An obstetrician accepted a diagnosis of pulmonary stenosis made 20 years previously and as the patient seemed well he did not refer her for reassessment or supervision. The antenatal course and delivery were uneventful but soon after delivery her condition deteriorated. She was found to have *transposition of the great ves-sels* and cardiac surgery was proposed but she died before this could be carried out.

These four cases once more underline the importance of full history tak-ing and clinical examination antenatally, and referral for expert advice even on suspicion of an abnormality.

A woman with *aortic stenosis* developed infective endocarditis and died undelivered at 30 weeks gestation.

This patient's care during pregnancy had been of poor quality. Although a cardiologist had been informed of her condition he had not proposed to see her unless her condition deteriorated, by which time it was too late.

The remaining death due to congenital heart disease was a woman who had had an *atrial septal defect* repaired. Pregnancy, labour and the puerperium were uneventful but 17 days after delivery she went swimming and died suddenly when she returned home. Autopsy showed endocardial fibroelastosis.

Acquired heart disease

There were nine deaths associated with acquired heart disease counted in this chapter. The diagnoses are listed in Table 11.2. In addition there was a death due to acute viral myocarditis which was regarded as *Fortuitous* and it is counted in Chapter 14.

Substandard care

Eight of the nine cases were judged to have had substandard care.

In four cases the patient had failed to heed strong advice against child-bearing:

> A poorly controlled diabetic refused admission for stabilisation. She developed left ventricular failure and died undelivered at 33 weeks gestation following a *myocardial infarct.*

> A diabetic woman with severe angina had extensive arterial disease and had had coronary bypass surgery and a renal transplant. She had been advised against pregnancy. She was delivered by Caesarean section at 35 weeks gestation because of fetal macrosomia. She died following *myocardial infarction* on the seventh post-partum day.

> A primigravida with *dilated cardiomyopathy* was advised against pregnancy. When pregnant she refused the offer of termination and died undelivered at 18 weeks gestation.

> An obese woman with *familial ß hyperlipidaemia, severe atheroma and hypertension* declined to stay in hospital in late pregnancy despite angina pectoris. She was readmitted in labour, had a spontaneous delivery and went home two days later. She was readmitted in cardiogenic shock and died 38 days postpartum. Autopsy showed 90% occlusion of the coronary arteries.

In four cases there were professional shortcomings:

> A woman who spoke little English failed to reveal that she had *mitral stenosis* and her GP did not inform the hospital of her cardiac history. Although a cardiac murmur was noted at the antenatal booking visit no action was taken. Her condition deteriorated and she had a Caesarean section. Immediate valve replacement was planned but her condition deteriorated further and she died the day after delivery before the cardiac operation could be performed.

> A recent immigrant primigravida was admitted with a spontaneous abortion at nine weeks gestation. She and her accompanying relatives failed to disclose that she had *mitral stenosis.* She developed septicaemia and acute myocarditis, from which she died the following day.

These two cases once more stress the importance of accurate history taking and examination especially when there are communication problems.

A woman with *dilated cardiomyopathy* had a bundle branch block and cardiac arrhythmia. She died suddenly, undelivered, at 15 weeks gestation.

In this case the seriousness of her condition had not been appreciated and therefore appropriate assistance had not been enlisted.

An older woman who was a heavy smoker was admitted at 31 weeks gestation with chest pain and extensive *myocardial infarction* was diagnosed. She responded to treatment and was discharged by the medical registrar six days later. Three days after this she was readmitted because of abdominal pain and diarrhoea. She had an antepartum haemorrhage and was delivered of a stillborn fetus. Her condition continued to deteriorate and a laparotomy was performed. There was extensive small bowel necrosis and she died on the second day after delivery. Autopsy confirmed that the bowel necrosis was due to mesenteric emboli from the myocardial mural thrombus.

Although the outcome would probably not have been different it was considered that it was unacceptable to send home a high risk woman in late pregnancy so soon after a major myocardial infarct and without adequate support and supervision.

The remaining death from acquired disease, in which there was not substandard care, was a woman delivered by Caesarean section because of fetal distress who developed *coronary ischaemia* at the time of the section and died immediately postpartum. Autopsy showed obstructed coronary flow due to an aneurysm.

Table 11.3   *Death from cardiac disease in relation to gestation*

	Congenital	Acquired	TOTAL
Aborted or died undelivered <30 weeks	1	3	4
Undelivered 30 weeks and over	-	1	1
During or within 24 hours of abour or Caesarean section	2	2	4
Up to 7 days postpartum	4	2	6
7 days or more postpartum	2	1	3
TOTAL	9	9	18

Time of death from cardiac disease

The time of death in relation to pregnancy is summarised in Table 11.3. The majority of deaths occurred during delivery or the first postpartum week and the importance of expert supervision and availability of support facilities at this time is stressed.

Comment

There was an unacceptable number of cases in which care was judged to be substandard. The reasons for substandard care vary but there are certain aspects which occur repeatedly and which should be emphasised.

In the seven cases in which the patient disregarded professional advice it was clear that the hazards of pregnancy were considerable and whilst the ultimate decision rests with the patient it is possible that techniques for advising women with life threatening conditions could be improved.

There is a need for more effective pre-pregnancy counselling of women with cardiac disease and, for women who still elect to become pregnant, expert supervision and combined care with a cardiologist.

The proportion of deaths due to congenital heart disease continues to rise and this group of patients seems particularly reluctant to accept medical advice concerning the dangers of childbearing.

High risk patients who are poor compliers and refuse admission to hospital need adequate domiciliary supervision and domestic support.

Deficiencies in history taking, clinical examination and assessment were common causes of substandard care and the potential seriousness of some conditions was not appreciated or was disregarded.

Reassessment of known cardiac disease in pregnancy by a cardiologist and assessment of patients in whom appparently minor symptoms or signs are detected on routine examination is imperative. Women with significant disease should have combined care.

CHAPTER 12

Other Indirect causes of maternal death

Summary

Ninety three *Indirect* deaths were recorded in this triennium, representing 34% of all Direct and *Indirect* deaths. This compares with 30% for the previous triennium. Eighteen deaths are described in other chapters and the remaining 75 deaths are discussed in this chapter.

There were eight reported *Late Indirect* deaths which are counted in Chapter 15: Six suicides associated with postnatal depression and two cases of carcinoma of the breast.

Definition

Indirect maternal deaths are defined as those resulting from a previously existing disease, or disease that developed during pregnancy, which did not have a *Direct* obstetric cause but which was aggravated by the physiological effects of pregnancy. Also included are deaths in which the pregnancy significantly affected the diagnosis, treatment or management of the associated disease (e.g. diabetes, epilepsy, appendicitis).

Causes of Death

The causes of death are summarised in Table 12.1.

Infectious diseases

There were six deaths related to infectious diseases, of which three were due to the complications of varicella and one each to malaria, aspergillosis and viral hepatitis

Varicella

> A woman in her thirties developed varicella at 21 weeks gestation. She was desperately ill at the time of admission and she was immediately transferred to the Intensive Therapy Unit where treatment with acyclovir and antibiotics was started. Termination of the pregnancy was planned but spontaneous abortion occurred.

Table 12.1 *Causes of Indirect deaths*

ICD9 CODE			Number of cases
001– 139	*Infectious diseases*		6
	Varicella	3	
	Malaria	1	
	Viral hepatitis	1	
	Aspergillosis	1	
140– 239.9	*Neoplastic diseases*		4
	Breast	2	
	Cervix	1	
	Other	1	
240– 279.9	*Endocrine, metabolic and immunity disorders*		5
	Diabetes mellitus	2	
	Phaeochromocytoma	1	
	Systemic lupus erythematosus	2	
280– 289.9	*Diseases of the blood*		1
	Idiopathic thrombocytopenic purpura	1	
430– 438	*Diseases of the central nervous system*		30
	Intracranial haemorrhage		
	Subarachnoid	12	
	Other	9	
345	Epilepsy	9	
440– 448	*Diseases of the circulatory system (exc. cardiac disease)*		4
	Ruptured splenic aneurysm	3	
	Aortic aneurysm	1	
480– 519.9	Diseases of the respiratory system		9
	Asthma	2	
	Pneumonia	4	
	Influenza pneumonitis	2	
	Bronchopulmonary sequestration	1	
540– 579	Diseases of the digestive system		3
	Appendicitis	2	
	Biliary cirrhosis	1	
580– 599.9	*Diseases of the genitourinary system*		2
	Post-operative haemorrhage	1	
	Glomerulonephritis	1	
E950– E959	*Sudden unnatural deaths*		
	Suicide		8
646.9	*Unexplained*		3
Total			75

Her condition continued to deteriorate and she was thought to have a staphylococcal pneumonia, although this was never confirmed bacteriologically. She developed the adult respiratory distress syndrome and lung transplant was being considered shortly before she died.

An elderly primigravida came from a family in which two other members had varicella. She was admitted as an emergency at 29 weeks gestation and died undelivered 12 hours later whilst acyclovir therapy was being considered.

A young para two caught varicella from her husband when she was 32 weeks pregnant. Treatment with acyclovir was initiated. She had a spontaneous premature delivery but subsequently developed streptococcal septicaemia, from which she succumbed.

There was no evidence of substandard care in any of these cases.

In the previous Report there were four deaths from the complications of varicella and the potentially serious consequences in pregnancy of a condition which is usually regarded as relatively mild require emphasis. Exposure to infected contacts should be avoided as much as possible and treatment with antivirals and antibiotics should be started early.

Malaria

An African, recently arrived in the United Kingdom, had a history of malaria which she did not reveal. She complained of 'aches and pains' at her last attendance at the antenatal clinic and was admitted four days later with rigors. Falciparum malaria was diagnosed at this stage. As soon as treatment had been started and her condition had been stabilised she was delivered by Caesarean section. She was treated in the ITU but on the third day postpartum she developed disseminated intravascular coagulation (DIC) and died seven days later.

Care was considered to be substandard because the patient had not been taking antimalarials, the history of malaria was not elicited and consequently the diagnosis was not considered when she attended the antenatal clinic. In any recently arrived patient from an endemic area who has a flu like illness malaria should be considered as a possible diagnosis.

Aspergillosis and asthma

A multigravida developed a 'flu like' illness at 22 weeks gestation and was admitted with severe asthma. She was diagnosed as having influenza A. Antibiotics, steroids and bronchodilators resulted in only temporary improvement. Spontaneous abortion occurred 12 days after admission. She remained pyrexial and aspergillosis was diagnosed on sputum examination but treatment with amphotericin produced no improvement. An autopsy was not performed.

Viral hepatitis

A recent immigrant was admitted to hospital at 24 weeks gestation because of drowsiness and jaundice. Liver failure was diagnosed, abortion was induced and she died three days later from non A, non B viral hepatitis. No autopsy was performed but immediate postmortem needle biopsy showed massive hepatic necrosis.

Neoplastic diseases

There were four deaths due to neoplastic disease.

Two women had carcinomatosis arising from primary breast disease. One died at 22 weeks gestation. The other had a mastectomy when 12 weeks pregnant but the disease progressed rapidly and she died 12 days after an emergency Caesarean section at 32 weeks gestation.

A primigravida was noted to have an 8cm ovarian cyst on routine ultrasound scan at 17 weeks gestation. She had a 'virus like' illness at 31 weeks gestation. Labour commenced prematurely at 33 weeks and an emergency Caesarean section was performed under epidural anaesthesia. The ovaries were reported as normal. At the time of delivery she was unwell, was cyanosed and had a swollen neck. In the puerperium she developed bilateral hydrothoraces and ascites but a firm diagnosis could not be made from aspirates. Her condition deteriorated and she died from carcinomatosis three weeks after delivery. Detailed autopsy and histological examination showed papillary adenocarcinoma which may have arisen from the ovary or pancreas. There was a 10cm ovarian cyst: histology showed a benign mucinous cystadenoma with papillary carcinomatous deposits on its surface.

A woman in her fourth decade had recurrent vaginal bleeding during pregnancy. Detailed investigation was deferred because of the pregnancy and she was ultimately found to have a carcinoma of the cervix.

Endocrine, metabolic and immunity disorders

Diabetes mellitus

There were two deaths from diabetes mellitus.

A poorly controlled diabetic was admitted as an emergency under a general surgeon at 28 weeks gestation with an axillary abscess.

She had severe keto-acidosis which failed to respond to treatment.

A young primigravida living alone had several admissions because of hypoglycaemia. At 25 weeks gestation she was found at home in coma. Soon after admission she aborted spontaneously. She failed to recover consciousness and died one month later.

In both cases there was poor patient cooperation and care was therefore substandard. In the first case it was considered that the medical care was also substandard in that there was delay in getting the advice of a medical team and further delay in admission to an intensive therapy unit because the first three units approached were full and unable to accept her.

Phaeochromocytoma

A woman in her thirties had been hypertensive during her pregnancy (maximum BP 160/100mm Hg). During Caesarean section for a transverse lie she developed ventricular tachycardia. A diagnosis of phaeochromocytoma was suspected and appropriate treatment initiated promptly but she failed to recover. The diagnosis was confirmed at autopsy.

In retrospect, there had been no specific clinical features, other than hypertension, to suggest the diagnosis before the crisis occurred.

Systemic lupus erythematosus

There were two deaths associated with systemic lupus erythematosus and in both cases there were elements of substandard care.

A young primigravida had persistent proteinuria. At 28 weeks gestation she became anaemic and there was evidence of haemolysis. Two weeks later she was admitted with a haemolytic uraemic syndrome and increasing joint pains, at which time she was found to have antinuclear antibodies. In spite of treatment with corticosteroids, antibiotics and blood transfusion her condition deteriorated. Whilst being transferred to a renal unit she had cardiac arrest and died.

Earlier more detailed investigation of the proteinuria in this case might have resulted in earlier treatment.

A woman on steroid therapy for systemic lupus erythematosus (SLE) had a history of pneumonia and septicaemia. She was delivered by Caesarean section under spinal anaesthesia because of fetal compromise at 34 weeks gestation. After delivery she was pyrexial and an SLE crisis was diagnosed. She improved with appropriate therapy but four days later she suddenly became desperately ill. A pulmonary embolism was suspected and she was transferred to the nearest intensive therapy unit, some ten miles away. Pulmonary embolism was excluded but idiopathic pulmonary hypertension was diagnosed. She died from cardio-respiratory failure.

This case again illustrates the problems of caring for a high risk patient in an isolated maternity unit remote from support facilities. However the fault was not in clinical judgment but in the organisation of the services in the area, there being no obstetric unit on a general hospital site with an intensive care unit.

Diseases of the blood

Idiopathic thrombocytopenic purpura

A multigravida with idiopathic thrombocytopenic purpura associated with antibodies to white blood cells and platelets was receiving prednisolone therapy. When she attended the antenatal clinic for booking at 17 weeks gestation she had multiple purpuric patches and was admitted to hospital. In spite of prednisolone 80mg daily and Sandoglobulin therapy her purpura failed to improve. Four days later she had a fit and remained in coma. CT scan showed a large intracerebral haemorrhage. Brain death was confirmed and life support was discontinued 24 hours later. Permission for an autopsy was refused.

Diseases of the central nervous system

Intracranial haemorrhage

There were 21 deaths from intracranial haemorrhage which are included in this section. In addition there were 12 deaths from cerebral haemorrhage in association with eclampsia or severe pre-eclampsia which are included in Chapter 2.

In seven cases the woman died undelivered and in four cases perimortem Caesarean section was carried out. Only two women had any symptoms prior to the fatal event. In 13 cases the diagnosis was confirmed by autopsy and/or surgery and in seven cases the only confirmation was from CT scan. In one case the diagnosis was based on clinical findings only. In three cases there was evidence of substandard care.

Subarachnoid haemorrhage

In addition to the 12 cases of subarachnoid haemorrhage counted here there were two cases associated with pregnancy related hypertension which are counted in Chapter 2.

Four women died undelivered. Three of these died suddenly at home and the fourth was comatose at the time of admission to hospital. Two other women were delivered by Caesarean section after brain death.

Table 12.2 *Deaths from intracranial haemorrhage*

		Number of cases
Subarachnoid haemorrhage		12
Confirmed by autopsy or surgery	9	
(Berry aneurysm found in 6 cases)		
Clinical +CT scan diagnosis only	3	
[Died undelivered	4]	
(+ 2 perimortem Caesarean sections)		
Other intracranial haemorrhage		9
Confirmed by autopsy	4	
(Origin not identified in any case)		
Clinical + CT scan diagnosis only	4	
Clinical diagnosis only	1	
[Died undelivered	3]	
(+2 perimortem Caesarean sections)		

A young multigravida collapsed at home at 39 weeks gestation. A diagnosis of subarachnoid haemorrhage was made by CT scan and she was transferred to the regional neurosurgical unit. Soon after arrival she had another massive haemorrhage. She was maintained on a ventilator and Caesarean section was performed with the birth of a surviving child. Life support was discontinued 48 hours later.

Apart from those who had perimortem Caesarean section four women died after delivery. Two had uneventful pregnancies and deliveries and died suddenly on the fourth and seventh puerperal days respectively. In the other two cases detailed below care was substandard.

A multigravida with a twin pregnancy complained of headaches and neck stiffness during the antenatal period and this necessitated her admission at 38 weeks gestation. Labour was induced with prostaglandin pessaries. During labour she had an epileptiform convulsion and her blood pressure rose to 220/125mm Hg. Spontaneous delivery occurred whilst preparations were being made for Caesarean section. She was treated with hydrallazine but had convulsions during labour. She had a massive postpartum haemorrhage requiring hysterectomy. Her circulatory state was stable but she failed to regain consciousness. She was transferred to the intensive therapy unit where she was declared 'brain stem dead' on the following day. A berry aneurysm was confirmed at autopsy.

It is probable that there had been previous episodes of subarachnoid bleeding and if the symptoms had been heeded surgical intervention might have influenced the prognosis.

> A young previously healthy primigravida had a convulsion during labour and an emergency Caesarean section was performed. She remained unconscious post-operatively. A consultant physician made a diagnosis of subarachnoid haemorrhage, which was confirmed by CT scan, but therapy was of no avail. A berry aneurysm was identified at autopsy.

There were delays in obtaining a consultant obstetrician, an anaesthetist and an opinion from a neurologist but it is unlikely that prompter action would have altered the outcome.

Other intracerebral haemorrhage

There were nine cases in which the origin of the intracranial haemorrhage was not determined. Three women died undelivered, having been admitted dead or in coma. In one of these cases autopsy established the diagnosis of intracerebral haemorrhage but no further detail was available and in the other two the diagnosis depended on CT scan. Perimortem Caesarean section was carried out in two cases.

Four women died soon after delivery.

> An older woman in her sixth pregnancy was an alcoholic with poorly controlled epilepsy. Labour was induced at 36 weeks gestation and she had a fit during labour from which she did not regain consciousness. A CT scan showed a left parieto-occipital intracerebral haemorrhage with possible arterio-venous malformation. No autopsy was performed.

> A young primipara developed drowsiness followed by fits six hours after a normal delivery. The diagnosis of intracerebral haemorrhage was confirmed by CT scan and she was first transferred to the ITU in another hospital and subsequently to the neurosurgical unit in a third hospital, where a craniotomy was performed. She died shortly afterwards.

This case again illustrates the problems of management of major emergencies in detached maternity units.

> A secundigravida had an uneventful spontaneous delivery. One and a half hours after delivery she complained of severe headache and vomited. Her blood pressure rose to 150/100mm Hg and she was given analgesics. Five hours later she was found unconscious in bed but failed to respond to resuscitation and was certified dead after a further five hours.

Care was considered substandard because of inadequate clinical observations and of the investigation and management of the symptoms.

One woman collapsed 12 hours after an uneventful twin delivery.

Epilepsy

There were nine deaths from epilepsy and its complications. Seven women died undelivered and in addition another woman had a postmortem Caesarean section. Two deaths were in early pregnancy, at eight and 13 weeks gestation respectively. One woman died two weeks postpartum but details were inadequate and there was no autopsy.

In at least eight cases there was substandard care (there was not sufficient detail to assess the ninth case) and it seems that the messages of previous Reports have not been heeded adequately. Epileptic patients often have other illnesses and many are poor compliers. One woman was also diabetic, one was asthmatic and another was an alcoholic. In five cases there was poor patient co-operation and more vigorous pursuit of these women might have improved their prospects. In only two cases was there a record of blood levels of anticonvulsants being measured antenatally; in one the assays were not sufficiently frequent and in the other a single assay was carried out after convulsions at 36 weeks gestation. There was insufficient collaboration between obstetricians and physicians in some cases. The need for cooperation and for careful assessment of needs and dosage of anticonvulsant therapy is again stressed.

A diabetic and epileptic woman in her twenties became pregnant against medical advice. She died suddenly from aspiration asphyxia when only eight weeks pregnant. It was not possible to determine whether epilepsy or hypoglycaemia was the primary event as she was unattended at the time of death and there were no postmortem drug assays.

A woman of low intelligence was asthmatic as well as epileptic. In spite of poor attendance the community staff made good efforts to maintain contact with her. Nevertheless there was poor communication between the medical staff, with the general practitioner in one district, the obstetrician in another and the neurologist in a third district. She was only seen once by the neurologist, at 18 weeks gestation, and he did not have her notes available. Although she had had convulsions no further investigations were undertaken and there were no anticonvulsant assays. At 38 weeks gestation she had a convulsion at home and died from asphyxia due to inhalation of vomit.

A young epileptic in her second pregnancy antenatally spent much of her time in hospital for primarily social reasons. She had a fit whilst in hospital and was seen by a medical registrar who advised no medication and allowed her to go home. At 35 weeks gestation she had a fit at home and died from aspiration asphyxia.

The medical care and supervision of this woman was considered to be substandard.

> A woman who had in the past had several admissions because of status epilepticus attended poorly during her second pregnancy in spite of repeated appointments with the obstetrician and the neurologist. At 32 weeks gestation she had a fit at home and, following a 999 call, the ambulance crew requested the attendance of the Obstetric Flying Squad. She was given intravenous Diazemuls but seven minutes later had respiratory and cardiac arrest. Endotracheal intubation failed. She was taken to the Accident and Emergency department at the nearest hospital where further resuscitation efforts were unsuccessful. After consultation with her husband postmortem Caesarean section was performed, at least one hour after the original cardiac arrest, and the baby was stillborn.

In this case a primary response by a paramedic ambulance team, if available, would have resulted in earlier expert resuscitative efforts, including cardiac defibrillation and this might have altered the outcome.

> An overweight alcoholic woman with poorly controlled epilepsy had become pregnant by donor insemination. She had epileptic fits throughout pregnancy. At 30 weeks gestation she was admitted moribund as the result of inhalation asphyxia following the onset of status epilepticus. Resuscitation was not possible.

Substandard aspects of her care included the doubtful advisability of assisted reproduction in such a high risk situation, poor compliance during pregnancy and long intervals between clinic visits and reviews of her therapy. Carbamazepine had been prescribed but none was present in post mortem blood samples, although low levels of phenytoin (which had not been prescribed) were detected.

Diseases of the circulatory system

Aneurysms

There were two deaths due to ruptured splenic aneurysm and another in which this was the presumed diagnosis. One death was due to rupture of a traumatic aortic aneurysm. In pregnancy these acute emergencies are often associated with problems of diagnosis and treatment.

Ruptured splenic aneurysm

> A primigravida was admitted shocked and in pain at 33 weeks gestation. The initial diagnosis was abruptio placentae. However

a scan showed free fluid in the peritoneal cavity and three hours after admission laparotomy revealed a ruptured splenic aneurysm and five litres of intraperitoneal blood. A Caesarean section was performed as soon as the bleeding was controlled but the baby was stillborn. Irreversible cardiac arrest occurred at the end of the procedure.

Care was substandard in that there was delay in diagnosis and consultant involvement and the initial resuscitative measures were inadequate.

A woman in labour in her third pregnancy complained of pain in her left shoulder and collapsed. It was thought that she had had an adverse reaction to pethidine and naloxone was administered. During the following 1½ hours her abdomen became distended and her haemoglobin concentration fell to 3 g/dl. By this time the baby was dead. Four litres of colloid were administered before blood became available. Three and a half hours after the initial collapse laparotomy revealed five litres of blood in the peritoneal cavity. A Caesarean section was performed to facilitate access but cardiac arrest occurred just before the spleen was removed. Resuscitative measures included thoracotomy and internal cardiac massage but there was no response.

A number of factors contributed to substandard care, including an inadequate and inappropriate response to the initial collapse, delay in getting expert help at several stages, inappropriate initial treatment because of an erroneous diagnosis, and the lack of donor blood on site resulting in excessive administration of colloid solutions and delay in surgery.

A young primigravida collapsed during labour. Intra-abdominal bleeding was suspected because of bruising in the groin. Resuscitation was started immediately by the consultant anaesthetist who was in the delivery unit and this was followed promptly by laparotomy which confirmed massive intraperitoneal bleeding. A stillborn infant was delivered by Caesarean section. By this time 11 units of blood had been given in addition to fresh frozen plasma and colloid. A consultant surgeon arrived promptly but had difficulty in identifying the source of the bleeding and death occurred during his exploration. The autopsy was of poor quality. There was a massive haematoma round the splenic artery but an aneurysm was not identified.

The clinical management of this case was exemplary throughout: Senior staff were in attendance from the outset, the diagnosis was made promptly and full resuscitation procedures were expertly applied. All necessary resources, including adequate supplies of blood, were available on site. Even so it was not possible to save the patient.

Post-traumatic aortic aneurysm

A woman who had previously suffered major trauma in a car accident developed acute chest pain at 38 weeks gestation. A diagnosis of thoracic aortic anaeurysm was confirmed radiologically. Her condition was stable and she was transferred 58 miles to the regional cardiac unit but collapsed shortly after arrival. Prompt attempts at resuscitation were unsuccessful. A Caesarean section was carried out on the spot but no paediatrician was present and no neonatal resuscitation equipment was available. The baby, weighing more than 3 kg, had an Apgar score of zero at one minute and died shortly afterwards.

Care was substandard in various respects although this almost certainly did not alter the outcome. Transfer of a seriously ill patient was made over a long distance without a doctor and without intravenous access. The obstetric team at the receiving hospital had not been notified and the cardiology registrar was unaware of the existence of an Obstetric Flying Squad. Resucitation had been attempted with the patient lying flat on her back.

Diseases of the respiratory system

There were nine deaths due to diseases of the respiratory system: two from asthma, four from pneumonia, two from influenzal pneumonitis and one from bronchopulmonary sequestration.

Asthma

A young woman who suffered from asthma and eczema had a ruptured ectopic gestation. Whilst being prepared for laparotomy she vomited, developed bronchospasm and respiratory and cardiac arrest. In spite of prompt response by the cardiac arrest team she could not be resuscitated. At postmortem examination there was only 200 ml of blood in the peritoneal cavity.

A woman in her thirties developed acute bronchospasm when setting out for hospital and was dead when the ambulance arrived. The records were not adequate to make any assessment.

Asthma was also a contributory factor in two other deaths, that due to aspergillosis, referred to above; and that due to influenzal pneumonitis, referred to below.

Pneumonia

In three of the four deaths from pneumonia there were elements of substandard care. Two of these are described below and the third is discussed in Chapter 9.

A gravida five had a spontaneous abortion at home whilst being treated for pneumonia. She had refused admission to hospital. She developed empyema, a tension pneumothorax and renal failure and was admitted to the ITU. Retained products of conception were evacuated but her condition deteriorated and she died 20 days after admission from adult respiratory distress syndrome.

Whilst this sequence of events was primarily due to the patient refusing advice it appeared that the general practitioner did not fully appreciate the seriousness of her condition.

A primigravida was admitted with suspected ruptured membranes and preterm labour at 30 weeks gestation. She was given ritodrine and corticosteroids and only retrospectively was a history of chest symptoms of four days duration elicited. Labour commenced the following day, by which time she had a productive cough and crepitations in the lungs. A forceps delivery was performed and she was given antibiotics intravenously. She developed septicaemic shock due to anaerobic streptococci and had fluid overload. She died on the 16th post partum day from adult respiratory distress syndrome.

Care was substandard because of delay in diagnosis which resulted in inappropriate medication for preterm labour, a factor which probably significantly affected her management, especially in relation to fluid overload, and the outcome.

An older woman had a breech delivery under epidural anaesthesia and was discharged apparently well on the fourth day. She was readmitted the following day with chest pain and it was not certain whether she had pneumonia or a pulmonary embolus, so she was treated with antibiotics and anticoagulants. A diagnosis of staphylococcal pneumonia was subsequently established. She developed adult respiratory distress syndrome and died four days later.

Influenzal pneumonitis

A young woman with severe kyphoscoliosis and asthma had a chest infection treated with antibiotics. She was admitted in labour with a breech presentation at 35 weeks gestation. It was only subsequently elicited that she had been unwell with respiratory symptoms in the preceding three days. She was delivered by Caesarean section under general anaesthesia. Immediately after the operation she developed bronchospasm and was pyrexial. A transbronchial lung biopsy caused bilateral pneumothoraces. In spite of appropriate treatment in the ITU her condition deteriorated and she required renal dialysis. She died from adult respiratory distress syndrome. Viral pneumonitis was confirmed by a rise in influenza A antibody titre and at autopsy.

Management decisions were clearly difficult in this case but there was delay in eliciting the respiratory history. Reassessment might have led to decision to allow vaginal delivery or to use regional rather than general anaesthesia. A consultant anaesthetist was not involved in this decision although it was clearly a high risk situation.

> A multigravida developed a chest infection at 35 weeks gestation and was treated by her general practitioner with antibiotics, salbutamol and steroids. She refused to stop smoking. Labour commenced spontaneously and was easy and uneventful. Post partum, in spite of intensive care, her condition deteriorated rapidly and influenza with aspergillosis was ultimately diagnosed. She developed adult respiratory distress syndrome and multiple organ failure and died 18 days after delivery.

Care fell short of desirable standards on a number of counts. The general practitioner apparently did not recognise the seriousness of her condition and it was considered that steroid therapy was inappropriate at that stage. The patient refused to stop smoking in spite of the seriousness of her condition. There was delay in making the bacteriological diagnosis because no service was available over the weekend.

Bronchopulmonary sequestration

> A young woman was known to have had a heart murmur in childhood and had pulmonary tuberculosis at the age of 19. She was seen at 18 weeks gestation by a cardiologist who diagnosed pulmonary hypertension. Her condition deteriorated as pregnancy progressed and she became dyspnoeic and cyanosed. At 36 weeks she developed severe pregnancy induced hypertension and was delivered by Caesarean section. She was treated in the intensive therapy unit but became pyrexial due to chest infection. It became increasingly difficult to maintain oxygenation and she died eight days after delivery. Death was ascribed to infection associated with bronchopulmonary sequestration. The sequestrated lower lobe of the left lung had anomalous arterial supply from the aorta and intercostal arteries which contributed to the pulmonary hypertension.

Diseases of the digestive system

Three deaths were due to diseases of the digestive system: two cases of appendicitis and one of biliary cirrhosis.

Appendicitis, peritonitis

> A non-English-speaking primigravida was admitted in late pregnancy with low abdominal pain and backache. Her condition improved and she was discharged after three days without a definite diagnosis. Three days later she had further abdominal pain

and vomiting but refused readmission. Four days after this she had a small vaginal haemorrhage; abruptio placentae was suspected but labour ensued. After delivery her abdomen was distended, the abdominal pain increased and bowel sounds diminished. Peritoneal aspiration revealed pus. Two days after delivery a laparotomy was performed. There was purulent peritonitis and a gangrenous appendix. Two further laparotomies were required to drain pus. On the 21st day, following tracheostomy obstruction, she had a cardiac arrest which responded to cardiac massage. A further laparotomy was planned but she died soon after the operation was started. Although the patient had refused readmission she was seen each day at home by a social worker who spoke her language.

A primigravida was admitted at 31 weeks gestation because of low abdominal pain. Initially she was thought to be in premature labour but appendicitis and urinary tract infection were considered. She was treated with antibiotics. Five days later ureteric obstruction was diagnosed and a percutaneous nephrostomy was attempted, unsuccesfully. By the seventh day after admission intrauterine fetal death occurred and spontaneous labour ensued. After delivery she developed septic shock and became moribund. A laparotomy was performed 12 hours postpartum and this revealed a perforated retrocaecal appendix, a large amount of intraperitoneal pus and gangrenous anterior abdominal wall muscle tissue. She failed to regain consciousness post-operatively.

These cases illustrate the problems of diagnosis of acute abdominal emergencies in pregnancy and the early puerperium. In the first case difficulties were compounded by the inability of the patient to speak English. Insufficient heed was paid to the symptoms in late pregnancy and immediately after delivery, leading to delay in diagnosis and surgical treatment. In the second case, although the diagnosis was considered initially it was over a week before the correct diagnosis was established, by which time the situation was hopeless. It was eight days from admission before the patient was seen by a consultant surgeon. Early consultation is essential when there is doubt about the diagnosis of abdominal pain in pregnancy in a clearly sick woman.

Biliary cirrhosis

A primigravida with primary biliary cirrhosis was considered fit for pregnancy by her gastroenterologist. At term she had an intrapartum haemorrhage and the baby was delivered with forceps. She collapsed after delivery, intraperitoneal haemorrhage was diagnosed and a laparotomy was performed. There was massive bleeding in the splenic area. It was not possible to ligate the bleeding vessels adequately. The abdomen was packed and 22 units of blood were transfused. She was transferred to a Liver Unit 30 miles away where a further laparotomy, together with splenectomy and hysterectomy were carried out. Cardiac arrest occurred during this procedure and she could not be resuscitated.

Failure to recognise gross splenic enlargement and portal hypertension antenatally led to failure to take adequate precautions and to make appropriate arrangements for delivery.

Diseases of the genitourinary system

Haemorrhage following nephrostomy for renal calculi

> A woman with renal calculi required postpartum percutaneous nephrostomy. On return to the ward she collapsed and was thought to have septicaemia. However her haemoglobin concentration fell rapidly to 3.4 g/dl and the diagnosis was revised to severe post-operative retroperitoneal haemorrhage. As preparations were being made for laparotomy cardiac arrest occurred. Cardiac output was restored temporarily, during which time the kidney was mobilised and the vascular pedicle was clamped. Cardiac output had again failed and in spite of open cardiac massage she could not be resuscitated.

There were two aspects of her care which were substandard but it is unlikely that either affected the outcome. There was possibly some delay in reaching the correct diagnosis and there were no beds available in the intensive therapy unit. However skilled staff and all necessary resuscitation equipment were available.

Glomerulonephritis

> A primigravida with type II mesangiocapillary glomerulonephritis who was in advanced renal failure had a spontaneous incomplete abortion. She was admitted to a hospital other than the one at which she was booked, evacuation of the uterus was carried out and she was discharged the same evening. Six days later her condition deteriorated and cardiac arrest occurred in the car whilst she was on her way to hospital. She had irreversible brain damage and died seven days later.

There was apparently serious communication failure in that the staff of the admitting hospital were not informed of her renal condition by the referring general practitioner and failed to elicit the history themselves. In consequence she was discharged too soon and adequate follow up arrangements were not made. However these shortcomings did not alter the ultimate prognosis.

Sudden unnatural deaths

Suicide

There were eight deaths by suicide counted in this chapter and in seven of these there was a history of mental disorder. Three women were known schizophrenics. In at least two cases there were deficiencies in management.

A schizophrenic woman on medication concealed her pregnancy. She had a normal delivery but her father refused to have her home. She was discharged to alternative accomodation on the eleventh day. She absconded a week later and two days after this was found in a house where she had hanged herself.

A woman suffered from depression during her second pregnancy. She became psychotic and had to be detained. She was admitted to the delivery unit for fetal monitoring at 38 weeks gestation but during a short period when she was not supervised she jumped from a high level window. A postmortem Caesarean section was carried out to try to save the child after an interval of about 15 minutes but the baby was already dead from multiple injuries.

Care was substandard in that there was inadequate supervision due to shortage of staff.

A young woman took a drug overdose during her third pregnancy. She recovered but refused follow-up. At 30 weeks gestation she killed herself by hanging. On arrival at hospital she was certified dead but as a fetal heart beat was reported a Caesarean section was carried out by the obstetric registrar approximately one hour after her death. The premature baby died soon after delivery.

There was a communication failure and the obstetricians were not informed of her psychiatric condition either by the psychiatrist (who only wrote concerning her admission after she was dead) or by the patient herself. A greater awareness might have helped to prevent her suicide.

In addition there were eight *Late* deaths from suicide associated with postnatal depression which are listed in Chapter 15.

Unexplained

There were three deaths without satisfactory explanation. All occurred in bed at night.

One woman was found dead in bed when 36 weeks pregnant. Although a presumptive diagnosis of viral myocarditis was made no specific cause for her death could be found in spite of extensive investigation.

The second woman was 18 weeks pregnant. She went to the toilet during the night, returned to bed and died suddenly ten minutes later. Autopsy showed severe pulmonary oedema for which a cause could not be found. Viral myocarditis was suspected but the autopsy was inadequate and provided no confirmatory evidence.

The third case was a woman in her thirties at 28 weeks gestation. She had a history of malaria but no recent problems. Her husband was achondroplastic and she was distressed having discovered that her fetus was also achondroplastic. She had a fit during the night, witnessed by her husband, inhaled vomit and died from asphyxia. Postmortem examination failed to reveal any cause for the fit. The only omission of relevance was a failure to perform any toxicological studies.

Comment

Pregnancies associated with medical and surgical disorders continue to be a major problem in obstetric practice and in a high proportion of cases there is substandard care. Although the diagnoses are diverse the deficiencies in management are similar.

There is often failure to recognise a disorder or to appreciate its significance in relation to pregnancy. This may arise because of poor history taking (sometimes compounded by language problems), inadequate clinical examination or failure to review a diagnosis which might have been made many years previously.

Management is often inadequate because of lack of appreciation of the effects of the physiological changes of pregnancy, such as haemodynamic factors, immunological status and altered drug metabolism, and lack of referral to and collaboration with appropriate specialists.

In all pregnant women with medical or surgical disorders consideration should be given to the best place for antenatal care and for delivery, ensuring proximity to intensive therapy or other specialist services relevant to the particular case.

As an emergency situation may arise at any time there should be adequate contingency plans which are clearly understood by staff on duty.

There is a need to improve professional advisory and counselling skills for women with pre-existing diseases, both before and during pregnancy.

CHAPTER 13

Caesarean section

Summary

Ninety one deaths followed Caesarean section. There were 60 *Direct* deaths, 24 *Indirect* deaths and seven *Fortuitous* deaths. In 12 of these cases the mother was close to death and receiving cardiopulmonary support; these 'perimortem' Caesarean sections are considered separately. In addition there were eight cases in which Caesarean section was carried out post mortem.

Excluding the peri- and post-mortem sections there were 57 *Direct*, 18 *Indirect* and four *Fortuitous* deaths in which delivery was by Caesarean section.

The steady fall in mortality associated with Caesarean section in England and Wales seen through previous triennia has not been maintained. In 21 cases care was judged to be substandard in relation to the management of the Caesarean section and/or associated after-care.

Seventeen *Late* deaths in which delivery had been by Caesarean section are counted in Chapter 15. In two of these cases the Caesarean section was relevant to the demise of the patient and these are described below.

During the years 1988–90 there were 91 deaths of women following Caesarean section, including 12 'perimortem' sections where the patient was terminally ill and receiving cardiopulmonary support, but excluding 8 postmortem sections. In Table 13.1 the perimortem cases for the last two triennia are included in the totals but are also shown in parentheses to facilitate comparison with previous Reports.

There was a rise in the number of *Direct* and *Indirect* deaths in women delivered by Caesarean section during this triennium (84 compared with 76 in 1985–87). Because of a change in the method of collecting hospital statistics and the non-availability of data it was not possible in the previous Report to estimate the number of Caesarean sections. For this Report data has become available for part of the triennium from hospital episode statistics and the number of Caesarean sections has been estimated from this to provide a denominator for the estimated fatality rates shown in Table 13.2.

TABLE 13.1 *Deaths connected with Caesarean section*, England and Wales 1973–90 and United Kingdom 1985–90*

		Total Maternal deaths	Direct deaths	Indirect deaths	Fortuitous deaths
England & Wales	1973–75	77	60	17**	
	1976–78	80	61	14	5
	1979–81	87	59	25	3
	1982–84	69	44	20	5
	1985–87	64 (9)#	42 (3)#	19 (5)#	3 (1)#
	1988–90	85 (10)#	58 (3)#	22 (5)#	5 (2)#
United Kingdom	1985–87	76 (11)#	50 (4)#	22 (6)#	4 (1)#
	1988–90	91 (12)#	60 (3)#	24 (6)#	7 (3)#

*   Postmortem Caesarean sections excluded.
**   Indirect and Fortuitous combined as Associated deaths for this triennium.
\#   Perimortem Caesarean sections included and shown in parentheses

Table 13.2 *Estimated number of Caesarean sections performed, and estimated fatality rate per thousand Caesarean sections within 42 days in NHS hospitals in England and Wales 1970–90 and the United Kingdom 1985–90*

	England & Wales	United Kingdom
Total maternities	2,087,442	2,360,309
Estimated Caesarean sections	228,413	278,500
Percentage of maternities by Caesarean section	10.9	11.8
Deaths after Caesarean section	85	91
Estimated fatality rate per thousand Caesarean sections	0.37	0.33

The estimated proportion of deliveries by Caesarean section has increased since the last available data (England and Wales 1982–84). The estimated fatality rate per 1000 sections for England and Wales (0.37) is the same as in 1982–84 but the United Kingdom figure is slightly lower (0.33).

Elective and Emergency operations

An analysis of the 75 *Direct* and *Indirect* deaths, excluding peri- and post-mortem Caesarean sections, related to elective and emergency procedures is given in Table 13.3. An *'unplanned emergency'* is defined as one where the need for operation overrides strict adherence to normal preparatory measures, such as a fasting period. This includes cases where elective Caesarean section had been planned but was pre-empted by clinical events. A *'planned emergency'* section is one in which appropriate preparatory care has been followed, including full assessment, fasting and the use of antacids.

Table 13.3   *Direct and Indirect deaths* related to elective and emergency procedures*

| | Deaths | | |
	Direct	*Indirect*	Total
Elective	19	8	27
Planned emergency	32	7	39
Unplanned emergency	6	3	9
Total	57	18	75

*Perimortem Caesarean sections excluded

There was a major reduction in the number of deaths following unplanned emergency operations from 21 to nine (from 34% to 12% of all Caesarean sections) suggesting that fewer hasty or inappropriate emergency decisions were being made.

Direct maternal deaths

The numbers of *Direct* deaths associated with Caesarean section by triennia for 1973–90 are shown in Table 13.4. There has been an increase since the last UK Report and for England and Wales the number is comparable with the triennia 1973–1981.

Table 13.4   *Direct maternal deaths within 42 days of Caesarean section*, England and Wales 1973–90 and the United Kingdom 1985–90*

	All *Direct* deaths	*Direct* deaths following Caesarean sections	Percentage of all *Direct* deaths	Caesarean section rate(%)	Estimated fatality rate/1000 Caesarean sections
England & Wales					
1973–75	227	60	26	5.63	0.59
1976–78	217	61	28	7.14	0.51
1979–81	178	59	33	8.9	0.35
1982–84	138	44	32	10.09	0.24
1985–87	121	42(3)#	35	N/A	N/A
1988–90	138	58(3)#	42	10.9	0.25
United Kingdom					
1985–87	139	50(4)#	36	N/A	N/A
1988–90	147	60(3)#	41	11.8	0.21

*   Postmortem Caesarean sections excluded in all triennia.

\#   Numbers and percentages in parentheses are perimortem Caesarean sections.

The principal indications for Caesarean section in cases of *Direct* maternal death are shown in Table 13.5.

Table 13.5 *Indications for Caesarean sections* in Direct maternal deaths United Kingdom 1988–90*

Indication	Elective CS	Planned Emergency CS	Unplanned Emergency CS	Total
Hypertensive disorders	3	8	4	15
'Fetal distress'		6	1	7
Protracted labour	1	4		5
Antepartum haemorrhage	4	8		12
Previous CS	3			3
Other obstetric indications	2	2		4
Other maternal indications	6	4	1	11
	19	32	6	57

*Peri- and postmortem Caesarean sections excluded

It is notable that there were no unplanned emergency operations associated with antepartum haemorrhage, i.e. in all cases there had been full assessment and preoperative preparation. There was also a reduction in the number of unplanned emergency operations for hypertensive disorders.

Indirect and Fortuitous deaths

There were 29 *Indirect* and 10 *Fortuitous* deaths and these are summarised in Table 13.6. In 16 cases the operation was performed peri- or postmortem and these are discussed later.

Immediate causes of death following Caesarean section

The attributed immediate causes of death following Caesarean section are shown in Table 13.7, with comparisons with previous triennia for the United Kingdom and England and Wales.

The greatest increase was in the number and the proportion of deaths from haemorrhage. The major reduction in anaesthetic related deaths seen in the last Report was maintained.

Table 13.6 *Causes of death in Indirect and Fortuitous deaths*

Cause of death	Number
Indirect deaths	
Malaria	1
Carcinoma of breast	1
Carcinoma cervix	1
Carcinomatosis	1
Phaeochromocytoma	1
Subarachnoid haemorrhage	1
Ruptured splenic aneurysm	2
Viral pneumonitis	1
Pulmonary hypertension	3
Bronchopulmonary sequestration	1
Other cardiac disease	5
Suicide	1
Perimortem sections	
Subarachnoid haemorrhage	2
Intracranial haemorrhage	2
Ruptured splenic aneurysm	1
Cardiac disease	1
Postmortem sections	
Epilepsy	1
Suicide	2
Ruptured aortic aneurysm	1
Fortuitous deaths	
Alcoholism	2
Carcinomatosis	1
Pneumonia	1
Perimortem sections	
Astrocytoma	1
Meningitis	2
Postmortem sections	
Road traffic accidents	3

Table 13.7   *The number and percentages (in parentheses) of all deaths after Caesarean section, including perimortem sections, classified according to immediate cause of death, England and Wales 1970–90 and United Kingdom 1985–90*

	Haemorrhage	Pulmonary embolus	Sepsis	Hypertensive disorders	Anaesthesia	Other Direct causes	Indirect and Fortuitous*	Total
England & Wales								
1973–75	8 (10)	6 (8)	8(10)	12(16)	17(22)	9(12)	17(22)	77
1976–78	8 (10)	9 (11)	8(10)	12(15)	18(22)	6 (8)	19(24)	80
1979–81	7 (8)	7 (8)	4 (5)	13(15)	19(22)	9(10)	28(32)	87
1982–84	4 (6)	12(17)	1(10)	10(14)	8(12)	9(13)	25(36)	69
1985–87	5 (8)	4 (6)	2 (3)	14(22)	3 (5)	14(22)	22(34)	64
1988–90	11(12)	12(14)	3 (3)	13(15)	3 (3)	16(18)	30(34)	88
United Kingdom								
1985–87	5 (7)	9 (12)*	2 (3)	14(18)	4 (5)	16(21)	26(34)	76
1988–90	11(12)	13(14)	4 (4)	13(14)	3 (3)	16(18)	31(34)	91

*Includes one death from arterial thrombosis

Peri- and postmortem Caesarean sections

Perimortem

The term *'perimortem Caesarean section'* was introduced in the last Report to identify cases in which cardio-respiratory support was used in virtu-ally dead mothers until a Caesarean section was performed, enabling delivery to take place in reasonably controlled conditions, usually by a consultant and with appropriate staff present. There were 12 such cases in this triennium. In most cases the patient was already in hospital and resuscitation was commenced very shortly after the initial collapse. Gestational ages ranged from 28 to 40 weeks. Three babies were lost and these cases are detailed below.

A laparotomy was performed on a collapsed woman with a rup-tured splenic aneurysm. The fetal heart had not been heard and Caesarean section was performed to afford access rather than for fetal considerations. The baby was stillborn.

A woman with an astrocytoma collapsed whilst in hospital. Intubation was performed immediately and the baby, weighing 3.9 kg, was delivered 37 minutes later in poor condition. There was difficulty with resuscitation and he died three days later.

A woman with meningitis was admitted unconscious when 37 weeks pregnant. Respiratory and cardiac arrest occurred soon after admission and resuscitation was commenced immediately. Cardiac arrest occurred several times whilst preparations were being made for Caesarean section. The baby weighed 3.4 kg and there was no difficulty in establishing respiration but early neonatal death occurred.

Nine perimortem Caesarean sections with successful fetal outcome were performed on mothers with: Intracranial haemorrhage(4), amniotic fluid embolus(2), meningitis(1), cardiomyopathy(1), acute fatty liver(1).

Postmortem

There were eight postmortem Caesarean sections, with no surviving babies. In most cases the operation had been done in hopeless and unsupported circumstances, without ready access to paediatric facilities. These cases included twins delivered at the roadside following a traffic accident; two deliveries approximately one and two hours respectively after maternal death in road accidents; and delivery of a dead baby with multiple injuries from a mother who had been dead for at least 15 minutes after jumping from a high building.

Late deaths

Seventeen *Late* deaths were reported in which delivery had been by Caesarean section. Factors associated with the Caesarean section were relevant in only two of the cases.

> A multigravida had a Caesarean section because of failure to progress in labour after two attempts at induction of labour for social reasons. Thirteen vaginal examinations had been performed. Blood loss was judged to be 'above average' but was almost certainly underestimated. The puerperium was stormy, with abdominal distension and pain, and a haemoglobin concentration of 6.6 g/dl. The patient was seen by a number of different doctors on succeeding days which probably contributed to delay in diagnosing peritonitis which was confirmed at laparotomy seven days postpartum. There were two litres of free pus in the peritoneal cavity and the uterus was grossly infected, with dehiscence of the scar and pus draining into the vagina. Subtotal hysterectomy was performed. A second laparotomy was required because of accumulation of pus and during this procedure the caecum was perforated. She became hypoglycaemic and developed cerebral infarction, resulting in coma from which she did not recover. She died seven months post partum.

Care was substandard in that there was delay in diagnosis of the peritonitis and failure to recognise the malfunction of a glucometer which led to non-recognition of hypoglycaemia.

> An obese woman had a Caesarean section because of severe hypertension. She had an associated clotting defect and was therefore not given prophylactic heparin. She could not be fitted with grad-

uated compression stockings because her legs were too fat. Postoperatively she had wound and chest infections but discharged herself prematurely. She died from a pulmonary embolus 80 days postpartum.

Care was judged to be substandard because of premature discharge from hospital against advice and lack of adequate follow up thereafter.

Substandard care

In 21 cases there was substandard care directly related to the Caesarean section and/or postoperative management. These are in addition to the *Late* deaths described above.

Availability of facilities and/or skills

In one case there was undue delay in obtaining blood products.

In 3 cases intensive care facilities were not available on site and this affected the quality of care available, to the detriment of the patient. In one case a seriously ill woman had to be transferred to an intensive therapy unit 35 miles away.

In another case there were inadequate facilities for the management of cardiac arrest.

In three cases there were problems in postoperative management to which inadequate staffing appeared to contribute. These included one case of airway obstruction, one case of respiratory depression and one case in which there was inadequate staff because of the number of patients being cared for at the time. In the latter case there was severe postpartum haemorrhage and the busy junior obstetrician could have summoned aid from the consultant but failed to do so.

In one case there was failure to diagnose Eisenmenger's syndrome preoperatively in a woman with antepartum haemorrhage.

In a woman with bleeding through pregnancy there was delay in diagnosing cervical carcinoma.

Inappropriate delegation

In seven cases there appeared to be inappropriate delegation of high risk cases to junior staff. Four repeat Caesarean sections were performed by unsupervised junior staff and they encountered problems beyond their skills. Five Caesarean sections for antepartum haemorrhage were delegated to registrars and in only one of these was there consultant supervision. In two cases of eclampsia and one of severe pre-eclampsia the operation and aftercare were delegated to registrars.

Inadequate consultation

In three cases the failure of junior staff to inform the consultant of problems resulted in substandard care which contributed to the demise of the patient. In a fourth case there was inadequate communication between the obstetricians and anaesthetists.

Other examples of substandard care in patients having Caesarean section but not directly related to the operation and postoperative care are mentioned in the appropriate chapters.

Comment

In spite of some welcome trends, including reductions in the number of unplanned emergency operations and of cases with substandard care the number of deaths associated with Caesarean section increased during this triennium.

The main immediate causes of death (as opposed to indication for operation) following Caesarean section were pulmonary embolus, hypertensive disease and haemorrhage, which together accounted for 41% cases. The large proportion of deaths associated with pulmonary embolism (14.3%) is a matter of concern and the place of prophylaxis requires further appraisal (See Chapters 4 and 17).

Many deaths, particularly from haemorrhage, were associated with inappropriate delegation of high risk cases, inadequate consultation and lack of adequate support facilities, all of which are amenable to correction.

Attention was drawn in the last Report to the poor fetal outcome in relation to postmortem Caesarean section. In this triennium there were eight such cases with no surviving babies. This again raises the question of the wisdom of hasty decisions and intervention in such cases, often made by junior staff without experience of these problems. In contrast there were 12 perimortem caesarean sections with uncompromised survival of nine infants. There were one stillbirth and two neonatal deaths but it was not possible to tell from the available data why the infants were lost as there was no clear evidence of prolonged maternal or fetal hypoxia in any of the three cases.

In the last Report it was emphasised that there is a need to have clear policies in relation to indications and circumstances for performing peri- and postmortem Caesarean sections. The decision to proceed to Caesarean section should be made at consultant level after careful assessment and preferably after discussion with the relatives.

CHAPTER 14

Fortuitous Deaths

Fortuitous deaths are those deaths which are unconnected with the pregnancy. These coincidental deaths are not considered as part of maternal mortality as internationally defined. The deaths are listed in table 14.1.

In 1988 to 1990 there were 39 *Fortuitous* deaths reported to the Enquiry, an increase of 13 cases compared to the previous triennium. In addition there were 25 *Late Fortuitous* deaths counted in Chapter 15.

AIDS

For the first time in the history of the Confidential Enquiries into Maternal Deaths an AIDS death is mentioned.

> The young primigravida was an immigrant from Africa whose pyrexial illness during pregnancy was diagnosed as sputum positive tuberculosis. Therapy was initiated and six weeks later she went into spontaneous labour at 34 weeks gestation. An apparently healthy infant was delivered. Subsequently pneumocystis carinii pneumonia was confirmed and HIV testing proved positive. Despite intravenous therapy with cotrimoxazole she died 14 days postpartum. The death was considered to be Fortuitous.

Neoplastic Diseases

In two cases the malignancy was thought to be the major pathology and the deaths were considered unrelated to the pregnancies

> An older primiparous woman miscarried at 15 weeks and died shortly afterwards from carcinomatosis secondary to primary breast carcinoma.

> A multiparous woman in her forties died suddenly at eight weeks gestation. Postmortem showed evidence of an earlier pulmonary embolism and a poorly differentiated adenocarcinoma of the ovary with omental secondaries.

Epilepsy

> A woefully incomplete Report form concerned a young woman whose sudden death in very early pregnancy was ascribed to epilepsy. She had a history of long-standing epilepsy.

The autopsy was considered inadequate as it did not include any clinical history, any organ weights, any histology report or any details of toxicology. The incidental pregnancy was discovered at autopsy.

Intracerebral Haemorrhage

Two women died from intracerebral haemorrhage.

A multiparous woman who was a heavy smoker had a spontaneous vaginal delivery of twins following induction of labour two weeks post term. Her blood pressure was 130/80mm Hg. She collapsed whilst visiting her babies soon after discharge and died two days later in the Intensive Therapy unit (ITU) from a massive intraventricular haemorrhage.

The other woman sustained a fatal cerebral haemorrhage ten days after delivery. She was normotensive and had also been delivered of twins without operative intervention.

It was considered that there were no avoidable obstetric factors in these two cases.

Influenzal Pneumonitis

A woman died from ARDS following influenza A infection. When her condition was failing she had a hysterotomy at 22 weeks gestation in an attempt to improve her respiratory function. Prior to the operation she was being ventilated and subsequently she developed renal failure and bilateral pneumothoraces. Autopsy was limited to examination of the thorax.

Asthma

Three women died from asthma.

One woman was 22 weeks gestation and had a long-standing history which included an acute attack requiring hospital admission two weeks prior to conception.

Another woman died from acute bronchospasm at home. This attack occured six days after an emergency Caesarean section which had been performed whilst she was deeply unconscious after she had taken an overdose of alcohol and benzodiazepines. During anaesthesia for the Caesarean section she had required intravenous aminophylline, salbutamol and hydrocortisone for bronchospasm.

The third woman, also a known asthmatic, suffered a fatal attack at 19 weeks gestation.

All three deaths were thought to be unrelated to the pregnancies.

Table14.1 *Fortuitous Deaths*

Causes of Death	Number
Infectious Diseases	
AIDS	1
Myocarditis of uncertain origin	1
Neoplastic Diseases	
Carcinoma of lung	1
Carcinoma of breast	1
Carcinoma of ovary	1
Cerebral glioma	3
Melanoma	1
Carcinomatosis ? primary	2
Retroperitoneal fibrosis	1
Blood Diseases	
Promyelocytic leukaemia	1
Diseases of Nervous System	
Meningoccal meningitis (Complement C 7 deficiency)	1
Pneumococcal meningitis	1
Streptococcal meningitis secondary to otitis media	1
Epilepsy	1
Diseases of the Circulatory System	
Intracerebral haemorrhage	2
Diseases of Respiratory System	
Asthma	3
Lobar pneumonia (non specific)	1
Post-influenzal pneumonia	1
Sudden unnatural deaths	
Fall - Head injury	1
Road Traffic Accident	8
Crush injury (from collapsing wall)	1
Accidental electrocution	1
Murder	1
Alcohol related	1
Burning (car fire)	1
Unexplained death *	1
TOTAL	39

*   This woman was found dead at home. Autopsy revealed a very early pregnancy but the cause of death was uncertain. The autopsy and the histology were poor. Although cardiomegaly had been mentioned the histology was not diagnostic of cardiomyopathy. The woman was grossly obese.

CHAPTER 15

Late Deaths

Deaths in women more than 42 days, but less than one year after pregnancy or delivery are defined as *Late* deaths.

A total of 48 *Late* deaths were reported in this triennium, and autopsies were performed in all but 15 of these cases.

In 1985 to 1987 only 16 *Late* deaths were reported to the United Kingdom Enquiry. This compared with 73 *Late* deaths for England and Wales alone in 1982 to 1984. This fall was due to a decision taken by the Assessors for England and Wales in 1984, that deaths over 42 days would be excluded from the 1985 to 1987 Report, in line with the current International Definition of Maternal Deaths (ICD9). However, it became apparent that strict adherence to this new rule was leading to the exclusion of a number of deaths which were related to pregnancy. For this Report it was decided that all deaths up to six months after pregnancy and delivery should be reported, and those deaths occurring between six and 12 months after pregnancy or delivery should be reported if Regional Assessors thought they were related to the pregnancy or delivery.

Scotland and Northern Ireland have continued to collect cases up to one year after pregnancy or delivery.

Late Deaths — Direct Obstetric Causes

Thirteen of the 48 *Late* deaths were considered to be directly related to maternal causes, despite the time which had elapsed since delivery.

Another death could not be confirmed as directly related.

> A young parous woman had asthma during her pregnancy and required steroids and ventolin. One week after delivery she was readmitted with right sided heart failure and she eventually died two months later from primary pulmonary hypertension.

Pulmonary thromboembolism could not be excluded as no autopsy was performed therefore this death was considered to be only indirectly related and is listed in table 15.1.

The following case histories detail the events related to the 13 maternal deaths with direct maternal antecedent factors.

> A multigravida had a forceps delivery for delay in the second stage. She inhaled gastric contents and died just outside the 42 day limit for the International Definition of Maternal Deaths.

The cause of death was given as Mendelson's Syndrome and her care was thought to be substandard. This case is discussed in Chapter 9.

In two cases death was associated with choriocarcinoma.

> A young primigravida died nine months after a normal delivery at term. Her presenting symptoms included chest pain, shortness of breath and malaise and at no stage during the four month period of her last illness did she report any gynaecological symptoms. During that time she was seen by a succession of seven locum general practitioners as it was the summer holiday season. Her investigations included two chest x-rays and a hospital admission, when she was diagnosed as suffering from atypical pneumonia. Autopsy revealed choriocarcinoma causing embolic occlusion of major pulmonary arteries. Unfortunately there was no histology of the uterus.

> An older primigravida had an uncomplicated spontaneous delivery at term. Eight months later she suffered repeated intracerebral haemorrhages and a rising beta hCG level led to the diagnosis of choriocarcinoma. Despite chemotherapy and partial removal of a right frontal tumour she had a further right occipital haemorrhage and died. Postmortem histology confirmed the presence of metastatic choriocarcinoma but histology of the uterus has not been forthcoming.

One exceptionally late maternal death occurred many months after a ruptured ectopic pregnancy, and although outside the remit of the Report has been included as an example of the relevance of reporting late deaths.

> The young woman sustained long standing and irreversible brain damage as a direct result of circulatory insufficiency following cardiac arrest which occurred during emergency surgery for a ruptured ectopic pregnancy. Three months after the initial event she remained unconscious and was developing quadriplegic spasticity. She was transferred to a rehabilitation setting for supportive care. She eventually died just over two years after her emergency operation.

Care was thought to be substandard in that there had been initial delay by the general practitioner and subsequent delay in obtaining an anaesthetist. It was also thought that there was failure to institute appropriate drug therapy in the event of an asystolic cardiac arrest.

Two women died from cardiomyopathy. The case histories will not be described here as this subject is commented on in Chapter 16.

Four women succumbed to pulmonary emboli.

> An obese multigravida with sickle trait had suffered a massive pulmonary embolism several weeks following an uneventful Caesarean section. She had a previous history of thrombophlebitis and suffered calf pain and pyrexia on the fifth day after Caesarean section. Despite this no anticoagulant therapy was instigated. She suffered a massive PE several weeks later.

> An obese hypertensive multigravida developed leg pain nine days postpartum and received a course of heparin for ten days. Four weeks later she suffered a pulmonary embolus and was treated with heparin and warfarin. Whilst still in hospital she had a cardiac arrest and died despite emergency pulmonary embolectomy.

There was delay in diagnosis and failure of communication between professional groups prior to her readmission. It was also thought that inadequate arrangements for acute life threatening emergencies contributed to substandard care following readmission to hospital.

> An obese woman collapsed 80 days after a Caesarean section at 38 weeks gestation when she had presented with fulminating pre-eclampsia. She had attended her GP only once ante-natally. This woman developed a post-operative chest infection. Prophylaxis for venous thrombosis was not carried out as she was thought to be too obese for graduated compression stockings and a clotting defect inhibited the use of subcutaneous heparin.

This was a high risk patient who was inadequately supervised pre- and postnatally, for which both the patient and her general practitioner were responsible.

> A woman in her thirties had a prostaglandin termination of pregnancy at 23 weeks following a intrauterine death. She developed a pulmonary embolism three weeks later and was discharged home on warfarin. Despite treatment she died some eight weeks after delivery. She was a heavy smoker and there was a family history of thrombosis.

The deaths of two women were related to pre-eclampsia:

> A young primigravida developed pre-eclampsia and had a planned emergency lower segment Caesarean section at 34 weeks

gestation performed by a registrar. Post-operatively she exhibited signs of continuing blood loss and a laparotomy revealed a huge haematoma in the utero-vesical pouch. Arterial bleeding from the uterine incision was controlled. She was cared for post-operatively in ITU but developed ARDS and died some seven weeks later. Consent for autopsy was refused.

Care was thought to be substandard because there was delay in diagnosing the initial haemorrhage and inappropriate haemodynamic management.

A young primigravida developed fulminating pre-eclampsia at 33 weeks gestation. Phenytoin was commenced and an epidural and central venous line were established before induction of labour by ARM and syntocinon. Following vaginal delivery, which occurred nine hours after induction, poor urine output and elevated central venous pressure were noted. Treatment with diuretics, human albumin and intravenous antibiotics was commenced. The woman developed disseminated intravascular coagulation and was transferred to a specialist renal unit. Initial improvement was not maintained and death occurred some eight weeks post partum in association with staphylococcal septicaemia, lung and kidney abscesses and ARDS.

It was concluded that the underlying cause of death was her fulminating pre-eclampsia. Antenatal care was thought to be substandard because her general practitioner delayed her admission and advised a week's bed rest despite proteinuria +++ and gross oedema and raised blood pressure.

Another death was due to septicaemia.

A young woman was admitted with a breast abscess three weeks after delivery. She had septic shock and died four weeks later. This case is also mentioned in Chapter 10.

Late Deaths — Indirect Obstetric Causes

There were ten cases where obstetric factors contributed indirectly to the death. They are listed in table 15.1. Cases in which there was a history of post natal depression are included here.

Late Deaths — Unrelated to Obstetric Causes

There were 25 such incidental deaths which are listed in table 15.2. Cases where there was a psychiatric history or a history of previous suicide attempts unrelated to pregnancy and no history of post-natal depression are included here.

Table 15.1 *Late Deaths - Indirect Causes*

Causes of Death	Number
Disease of circulatory system	
Primary pulmonary hypertension	1
Neoplastic Disease	
Carcinoma of breast	2
Sudden unnatural deaths — Suicide	
Insulin overdose following stillbirth	1
Mixed drug overdose following stillbirth	1
Amitryptilline. Post-natal depression	1
Hanging. Post-natal depression	2
Set fire to herself. Post-natal depression	1
Iatrogenic	
Hypoglycaemia during prolonged intubation after CS followed by peritonitis*	1
Total	10

*   See Chapter 13 for details.

Table 15.2   *Late Deaths — Unrelated to Obstetric Causes*

Causes of Death	Number
Infectious Diseases	
Streptococcal septicaemia	1
? Mumps	1
Septicaemia unspecified	1
Neoplastic Diseases	
Melanoma	1
Leukaemia	1
Carcinomatosis. Pulmonary carcinoma	1
Carcinomatosis. Carcinoma of stomach	1
Medulloblastoma	1
Carcinoma of ovary*	2
Carcinoma of bile duct	1
Carcinoma of breast**	1
Diseases of the Circulatory System	
Cerebral Infarction	1
Myocardial Infarction	1
Rheumatic heart disease	1
Sub arachnoid haemorrhage	1
Post-operative haemorrhage	1
Infective endocarditis	1
Cerebral haemorrhage due to A/V malformation	1
Diseases of Nervous System	
Epilepsy (drowned in bath)	1
Meningoccocal meningitis	1
Unexplained Deaths	
Drowning (open verdict)	1
Sudden Unnatural Deaths	
Suicide (cut throat)	1
Overdose with Co-proxamol tablets	1
Fall (? alcohol related). Head injury	1
Total	25

* Squamous carcinoma in ovarian dermoid	1
Mucin-secreting carcinoma	1

** This death was classified as Fortuitous, not Indirect, as the woman died two months after an 8 week gestation TOP operation performed because of her advanced malignancy.

CHAPTER 16

Pathology

Summary

Of the 325 deaths reported in this triennium autopsies were performed on 265 (82%). The autopsy and report were considered adequate in 208 (78%) but only 91 (34%) were of the high standard
expected by the Confidential Enquiry. Histology was performed on
176 (66%) of the autopsies and in one case there was a postmortem
needle biopsy of the liver without autopsy. In only 124 cases was the
histology report considered adequate.

The quality of the autopsy

The standard of the autopsies was similar to that in the previous
report. It is disappointing that there were still many substandard
reports which did not provide the detailed information which the
Confidential Enquiry required for its investigation. The major criticism
of the 57 unsatisfactory reports was the brevity of the description of the
organs, frequently omitting organ weights which provide a more objec-
tive measurement of mass. The worst example was where the report provided only a cause of death without any description of the autopsy findings

Autopsies performed at the request of HM Coroners/Procurators Fiscal

The great majority of autopsies in the review (90%) were performed on
the instruction of HM Coroners/Procurators Fiscal. In one case the coroner
authorised the removal of organs for donation but refused permission for
autopsy. This was unfortunate as examination of the brain for superior
sagittal sinus thrombosis would have been valuable.

It continues to be a matter of concern that some Coroners are only prepared to authorise further microbiological, histological or toxicological
examination if it is considered necessary to hold an inquest. Because of
this restriction information which would have been of value to the
Confidential Enquiry has been lost. It must be emphasised again that in
all cases of *Direct* and *Indirect* maternal death appropriate further examination should be undertaken as a matter of routine. Pathologists should
discuss this requirement with Coroners/Procurators Fiscal and, if necessary, with their Health Authorities/Boards/Trusts so that necessary
financial arrangements can be made. If required, local consultant obstetricians should be asked to provide their support in seeking satisfactory
arrangements for these autopsies.

Table 16.1 *Subjective assessment of the adequacy of autopsies in Direct maternal deaths 1988–90, United Kingdom*

Chapter	Total Deaths	Autopsies			Histology	
		None	Satis	Unsatis	Satis	Unsatis/ no record
Hypertensive disorders of pregnancy	27	5	17	5	11	11
Antepartum and post- partum haemorrhage	22	1	14	7	11	10
Thrombosis and thromboembolism						
Pulmonary embolism	24	2	18	4	11	11
Cerebral venous thrombosis	6	1	4	1	1	4
Cerebral arterial thrombosis	3	2	1	0	1	0
Amniotic fluid embolism	11	0	8	3	4	7
Early pregnancy deaths						
Ectopic pregnancy	15	0	10	5	3	12
Abortion	3	0	2	1	1	2
Genital tract sepsis	13	1	9	3	5	7
Genital tract trauma	3	0	3	0	0	3
Deaths associated with anaesthesia	4	0	4	0	4	0
Other *Direct* deaths	14	2	11	1	8	4
Late deaths	13	0	9	4	8	5
Totals	158	14	110	34	68	76

Note: Histology reports listed as unsatis/no record do not include patients on whom an autopsy was not performed.

Table 16.2 *Subjective assessment of the adequacy of autopsies in Indirect maternal deaths 1988-90, United Kingdom*

Chapter	Total Deaths	Autopsies			Histology	
		None	Satis	Unsatis	Satis	Unsatis/ no record
Infectious diseases	6	1	4	1	1	4
Neoplastic diseases	4	2	2	0	2	0
Endocrine and metabolic disorders and immune disorders	5	0	4	1	3	2
Blood diseases	1	1	0	0	0	0
Diseases of the central nervous system	30	6	18	6	12	12
Diseases of the circulatory system						
Aneurysms	4	0	3	1	2	2
Cardiac disease	18	5	9	4	5	8
Diseases of the respiratory system	9	1	8	0	6	2
Other Indirect deaths	8	1	6	1	5	2
Sudden unnatural deaths	8	0	7	1	1	7
Late deaths	10	5	5	0	1	4
Totals	103	22	66	15	38	43

Note: Histology reports listed as unsatis/no record do not include patients on whom an autopsy was not performed. The figures do not include 64 *Fortuitous* deaths.

Infections

There were 48 cases in which infection, other than terminal bronchopneumonia, was given as the cause of death. Of these, the diagnosis of infection was based on antemortem culture, serology or histology in 19 cases, postmortem culture in 16 and in three cases there was both antemortem and postmortem culture. In 17 cases there was postmortem histological evidence of infection/inflammation but in seven cases the histological report was inadequate. In nine of the 48 cases there was no microbiological or histological examination to confirm infection. However, the diagnosis of infection in one of these cases was based on the operative findings of an appendix abscess and in three cases the diagnosis of varicella pneumonitis was based on the clinical diagnosis of chickenpox. No lung histology was examined in these three cases. In five cases the diagnosis of infection given on the death certificate could not be substantiated.

Hypertension

There were 27 deaths directly attributed to hypertensive disorders of pregnancy in this triennium. Autopsies were performed on 22 cases, of which ten were of a high standard. Histology was not performed on three of the 22 cases and in a further eight cases the histology report was inadequate, most commonly because of a lack of histology on organs such as the liver and kidney which are important for showing features of severe pre-eclampsia/eclampsia. Adult respiratory distress syndrome (ARDS) was diagnosed in ten cases of which eight were confirmed at autopsy. Fifteen cases were associated with intracranial pathology, two subarachnoid haemorrhage, 11 intracerebral haemorrhage, one brain stem infarction and one cerebral oedema. In three of these cases there was no autopsy; in two the diagnosis was based on CT scan (one cerebral oedema, one cerebral haemorrhage) and the third (diffuse subarachnoid haemorrhage) by CT scan and lumbar puncture in a neurosurgical unit.

In addition to these 27 cases there were 17 deaths where hypertensive disorders of pregnancy were present but were not classified as the direct cause of health. In nine of these cases Caesarean section had been performed, of which six developed post-operative infection. Additionally, one case following surgical rupture of the membranes developed infection. The immediate cause of death in these seven infected cases was disseminated intravascular coagulation (DIC) complicating septicaemia (2), ARDS complicating septicaemia (4) of which two were *Late* deaths, and Gram negative septicaemia complicating uterine cellulitis (1). Of the remaining ten cases in this group there were four cases of ARDS, one amniotic fluid embolism, one pulmonary thromboembolism, one cerebral haemorrhage and three subarachnoid haemorrhage due to ruptured berry aneurysms. Autopsies were performed on all but one of these cases and in only two was the report substandard. There was a histological report on 13 cases in two of which it was inadequate because sections had not been examined for features of pre-eclampsia/eclampsia.

Haemorrhage

There were 22 cases where death was due to antepartum or postpartum haemorrhage. Autopsies were performed on all but one of these cases. In eight the autopsy report was of a high standard but in seven the autopsy report was inadequate or missing. The main criticism was the inadequate description of the genital tract and of the possible source of haemorrhage. In six cases hysterectomy had been performed in an attempt to control bleeding but in none of these was there a description of the uterus attached to the autopsy report.

In ten of the autopsy cases postmortem histology was inadequate or had not been performed. In one further case, where there was no autopsy, there had been a postmortem needle biopsy of the liver. In ten cases there was clinical evidence of DIC and this was confirmed by histology in six. In one case bleeding was thought to have arisen from a cervical laceration but at autopsy there was a poor description of the genital tract and there was no comment about the cervical trauma.

Although it may be difficult at autopsy to identify the source of even massive haemorrhage there should always be a detailed description of the genital tract including, if appropriate, a hysterectomy specimen. Particular care should be taken in looking for evidence of genital tract trauma and there should always be a comment about the placental site. Many of these cases develop DIC which may be the cause of or contribute to the fatal haemorrhage. Evidence of a thrombotic coagulopathy should be sought by histological examination of a wide variety of tissues especially the kidneys, adrenals and lungs. Likewise it is essential to look for evidence of amniotic fluid embolism which may have precipitated the DIC.

Pulmonary thromboembolism

Pulmonary embolism continues to be one of the commoner causes of maternal death. At autopsy, information on the source of the emboli, especially whether from pelvic veins or deep veins of the leg, should be sought.

In this triennium there were 24 deaths due to pulmonary thromboembolism. Additionally, there were eight cases where pulmonary embolism contributed to death, three associated with carcinomatosis (two carcinoma of ovary, one carcinoma of lung), one abruptio placentae, one anaesthetic death and three other *Late* deaths.

Of the 24 *Direct* deaths, autopsies were performed on 22. In the two cases without autopsy, pulmonary embolectomy was performed on one and, in another a venogram, initially reported as negative for deep vein thrombosis of the legs, was subsequently interpreted as positive. In each of the 22 autopsies embolus was found in the pulmonary trunk or branches of the pulmonary artery. In ten cases the source of the embolus was not identified but in a further nine cases there was deep vein thrombosis in the legs and in three cases there was pelvic vein thrombosis. In one of these cases both the deep veins of the leg and the pelvic veins were thrombosed. In a further case thrombus was found in the inferior vena cava but there was no comment in the report on the pelvic or leg veins. This case was unusual in that amniotic fluid embolism was also identified.

> A woman in her forties had a prostaglandin induction at 41 weeks following an intrauterine death. Two weeks later she complained of abdominal pain; ultrasound examination revealed a cystic area in the right adnexa. At laparotomy a haemorrhagic mass was found in the retroperitoneal tissues extending into the broad ligament and mesosalpinx. The patient died on the operating table. Autopsy revealed multiple pulmonary throemboli and thrombus in the inferior vena cava. Histological examination was reported as showing amniotic squames and lanugo hair in veins of the parametrium but no fetal tissues in the pulmonary thromboemboli.

Although amniotic fluid embolism may be found in the pelvic veins its presence in this case two weeks after delivery without evidence of amniotic fluid in the pulmonary vasculature was remarkable. Although bleeding had occurred into the retroperitoneum there was no evidence of disseminated intravascular coagulation.

Cerebral venous thrombosis

There were six deaths attributed to cerebral venous sinus thrombosis and a further four of cerebral infarction, of which one was a *Late* death. In the six cases of venous sinus thrombosis autopsies were performed on five. In four of these cases the brain was submitted for neuropathological examination and in all four there was a detailed report of the macroscopic findings by the neuropathologist; histological examination of the brain was performed on only one case. The fifth case was not examined by a neuropathologist, nevertheless the macroscopic description was satisfactory although here again there was no histological examination on the brain. In two of these five cases thrombosis of the superior sagittal sinus was demonstrated.

> In a third case streptokinase had been injected into the superior sagittal sinus and in this case thrombus was demonstrated in the right lateral (transverse) and sigmoid sinuses extending into the internal jugular vein. There were also small pulmonary thromboemboli apparently arising from the internal jugular vein.

In the remaining two autopsy cases thrombosis was described in the superficial veins of the brain. In one of these cases there was meningitis but the superior sagittal sinus was not submitted to the neuropathologist for examination nor was the cerebrospinal fluid cultured. In the other case, although venous sinus thrombosis was reported there was no detail of the site of this thrombosis.

In the case which did not come to autopsy CT scan during life was diagnosed as superior sagittal sinus thrombosis with diffuse cortical oedema. The major organs were removed for donation in this case but authority for autopsy was withheld.

Cerebral infarction

Only one of the four cases diagnosed as cerebral infarction came to postmortem examination. In this case there was infarction associated with left middle cerebral artery thrombosis. Two of the remaining cases were receiving heparin because of a preceding deep vein thrombosis in the legs. CT scan in one was described as showing cerebral infarction for which a cause could not be found. In the other, the infarct was in the distribution of the anterior and middle cerebral arteries. CT scan revealed thrombosis of the left internal carotid artery. The fourth case, a *Late* death, had a massive cerebral infarct, revealed by CT scan, in the distribution of the left middle cerebral artery four months after delivery of a term baby.

Amniotic fluid embolism

As in previous reports the diagnosis of amniotic fluid embolism required the histological confirmation of amniotic fluid in the maternal circulation. There were 11 cases where this criterion was met.

In a further five cases the possibility of amniotic fluid embolism had been considered before death but could not be confirmed at autopsy in four and because there was no autopsy in the fifth case.

In another four cases, although products of conception were reported in the maternal circulation it was concluded that the main cause of death could not be established as amniotic fluid embolism. One of these has been described above where it was concluded that death was due to pulmonary thromboembolism.

> The second case was a young woman who was delivered of a live baby after a spontaneous labour at 37 weeks. Although she had been normotensive before delivery she complained of a headache one hour after delivery when her blood pressure had risen to 170/90mm Hg and she had albuminuria. She had a grand mal seizure. A subarachnoid haemorrhage was suspected but not confirmed; a brain scan was negative. She developed renal failure and died a few days later. It was concluded that death was due to postpartum eclampsia. The autopsy and histology were of poor quality. The changes of ARDS were present in the lungs but positivity for keratinised squames in the maternal circulation was also queried.

> The third case had labour induced but fetal distress occurred and forceps were applied before full cervical dilatation. The cervix was lacerated and there was massive postpartum haemorrhage which appeared to be coming from the cervix. The bleeding was complicated by (DIC) from which the patient died. The autopsy and histology were of poor quality. The histological report mentioned a placental embolus rather than amniotic fluid embolus in the maternal pulmonary artery but the histological sections were not available for review.

> The fourth case had a history of repeated abortions. A cervical suture was inserted at 14 weeks. At 21 weeks she was admitted with spontaneous rupture of the membranes. She was pyrexial but a high vaginal swab grew commensals only. Two days later she collapsed and was thought to be in septicaemic shock. She developed DIC followed by cardiac arrest. Although the autopsy report was of a high standard the histology was inadequate. There was a purulent placentitis but no culture was reported. The urine grew *Escherichia coli*. The histology report made a suggestion of amniotic fluid embolism in the maternal pulmonary vasculature but this was poorly described and open to doubt. It was concluded that death was due to septicaemia.

It is important that the histological diagnosis of amniotic fluid embolism is firmly established. It is not satisfactory to describe features 'suggestive of' or 'compatible with' fetal squames if special techniques using immunohistological stains for cytokeratins or special stains for mucin and fat have not been applied. The sensitivity of detection of amniotic fluid embolism can be increased by using the buffy coat of pulmonary arterial blood.

Genital tract trauma

There were three cases where death was directly attributed to genital tract trauma, two of spontaneous uterine rupture and the third of traumatic rupture associated with forceps delivery. In all three cases autopsies were performed and these were considered adequate in two and of high standard in the third. In two cases hysterectomy had been performed in an attempt to control bleeding. The pathologist ensured that the excised specimens were examined and revealed transmural tears, one through a Caesarean section scar. Although the internal iliac arteries had been ligated in one of these cases the internal iliac vein was torn and massive bleeding occurred. The pathologist failed to demonstrate the trauma to this large vessel. In the third case the uterus was examined at autopsy in situ.

In only one of these cases was there a histological report and in this case histology was limited to the uterus. Postmortem histology is an important part of the investigation of spontaneous uterine rupture and failure to examine the uterus histologically in two of these cases is considered substandard.

In a further three cases genital tract trauma was considered to have contributed to death. Although autopsies were performed on all three cases it was inadequate in one.

> In this case there had been laceration of the broad ligament in the course of Caesarean section. Ligation of the broad ligament and hysterectomy were performed but the uterus was not later examined. The description of the genital tract and pelvic vasculature was poor. Clinically it was thought that DIC may have contributed to the bleeding but at autopsy no histology was taken to look for evidence of DIC.

In only one of these three cases was there histological examination and this, together with the autopsy report, were of a high standard.

Cardiac disease

There were 23 deaths associated with cardiac disease in this triennium. Of these four were *Late* deaths and one was *Fortuitous*. All of the remaining 18 were considered to be *Indirect* deaths.

Late cardiac deaths

Of the four *Late* deaths one was attributed to myocardial infarction, one to thrombosis of a mitral valve prosthesis following postpartum mitral valvotomy and two to dilated cardiomyopathy. In three of these cases the autopsy report was considered adequate but in only two, the cases of dilated cardiomyopathy, was there histology.

> The first of these cases of dilated cardiomyopathy was a woman who developed pre-eclampsia and was delivered by Caesarean section at 39 weeks. The following day she had intermittent dyspnoea and bronchospasm diagnosed as left ventricular failure. She was discharged five weeks later but readmitted after a further two weeks when she was diagnosed by echocardiography as suffering from dilated cardiomyopathy. She died in congestive cardiac failure 11 weeks postpartum.

The autopsy report was inadequate and although a large heart was mentioned it was not possible on review to make an accurate assessment of size as the weight of the heart was not recorded. Histological sections of the myocardium were reviewed by an experienced cardiac pathologist who considered the changes were compatible with the clinical diagnosis.

This case exemplifies the need for detailed autopsy descriptions of major organs, including their weights, with accompanying histology even in these *Late* maternal deaths.

> The second case, a young woman, developed nocturnal dyspnoea two weeks after a term delivery. Her initial treatment for cardiac failure was successful but she then suddenly collapsed and died. Autopsy demonstrated features of a dilated cardiomyopathy. Histology revealed a little lymphocytic infiltration of the myocardium and focal necrosis but culture of the myocardium and blood for viral antibody titres revealed no evidence of infection.

In all such cases it is important that microbiological evidence of infection is looked for. Histological examination of several areas of the myocardium including both ventricles and the septum should be undertaken to look for features of myocarditis.

Cardiomyopathy

In the context of this maternal death enquiry only cases of so-called primary cardiomyopathy are included. There were five deaths clinically thought to be due to cardiomyopathy, including the two *Late* deaths already described. Another case of dilated cardiomyopathy was unusual in the early onset of the disease in pregnancy.

> This young woman developed signs of cardiac failure with arrythmia and hypotension at nine weeks gestation. Six weeks later she

collapsed and died suddenly. At autopsy a grossly enlarged and dilated heart weighing more than 50% above the normal upper limit was found. Myocarditis was not confirmed in the adequate histological report. No virological studies were undertaken.

Another woman with dilated cardiomyopathy had suffered from this disease for four years before her sudden death at 18 weeks gestation in her first pregnancy. This autopsy provided a full detailed report of the heart and great vessels.

There was one case of hypertrophic cardiomyopathy in which there was a strong family history of this disease.

In two additional cases the diagnosis of cardiomyopathy could not be substantiated.

The first case was a grossly obese woman found dead. At autopsy there was a very early pregnancy. The autopsy report was inadequate but a moderately enlarged heart was described. Histology of the heart revealed a few hypertrophic myocardial fibres. This was considered inadequate evidence of a cardiomyopathy and the death has been classified as unexplained.

The second woman was delivered at 33 weeks after artificial rupture of the membranes for fulminating pre-eclampsia. Postpartum she developed *Staphylococcus aureus* septicaemia with hepato-renal failure. Because her heart appeared enlarged she was diagnosed as having a dilated cardiomyopathy from which she was thought to have died nine weeks postpartum. At autopsy the heart was dilated but only marginally increased in weight. There were bilateral lung abscesses and changes of ARDS in the lungs. It was concluded that she had died of septicaemia complicated by ARDS.

Congenital heart disease

There were eight cases of congenital heart disease excluding the case of familiar hypertrophic cardiomyopathy already mentioned — two of primary pulmonary hypertension, two atrial septal defects, one patent ductus arteriosus, one Fallot's tetralogy, one aortic stenosis and one transposition of the left and right ventricles. There was no autopsy in three of these cases. In the remaining five the autopsy report was of a high standard in two and adequate in another two. In one case the report was inadequate.

This case of aortic stenosis due to a congenital bicuspid aortic valve showed vegetations on the damaged valve. No culture was taken and there was no histology although there was evidence of embolisation from the vegetations.

This case demonstrates the failure of the autopsy to establish that the vegetations were due to infective endocarditis although this remains the probable diagnosis.

Histology was performed on only one case and here it was of a high standard. In another case a macroscopic diagnosis of endocardial fibro-elastosis was not confirmed because of the lack of histology.

Rheumatic heart disease

There were three cases of mitral valve disease two of which required mitral valvotomy. One of these was a *Late* death six months after delivery. No autopsy was performed on one of these cases and in the other two the autopsy reports were substandard. In neither case was there a histological report.

Cardiac disease remains one for the commoner causes of maternal death. The inadequacy of many of the autopsy reports emphasises the need for detailed descriptions of the heart including the total weight and, if appropriate, also the weights of the isolated right and left ventricles. Where infection is suspected adequate samples should be taken for bacteriological and virological studies. There should be accompanying histology in all cases.

Epilepsy

There were ten cases where the cause of death was given as epilepsy. In one of these cases epilepsy could not be confirmed and the death is classified as unexplained. Although doses of anticonvulsant drugs necessary to maintain therapeutic blood levels need to be increased in pregnancy, in only three of these ten cases was measurement of anticonvulsant drugs in postmortem blood estimated to assess compliance and adequate therapy. In all such cases blood for toxicology should be collected.

Aneurysms

There were 14 deaths associated with aneurysms in this triennium. Of these, nine were berry aneurysms on the circle of Willis or more distal major cerebral arteries. Eight were found at autopsy and one was diagnosed by CT scan.

There was one ruptured calcified aneurysm on the intracranial segment of the internal carotid artery which was diagnosed radiologically but there was no autopsy. This case is counted under subarachnoid haemorrhage. Two deaths were due to ruptured splenic aneurysms, one due to a ruptured thoracic aortic aneurysm in which there was a history of a severe road traffic accident in the past, with chest injuries. In this case it was thought that the aneurysm may have been related to the previous trauma. In one case there was an aneurysm at the bifurcation of the left coronary artery leading to arterial occlusion. This case is counted under cardiac deaths.

In addition to these 14 cases there were six where haemorrhage may have been due to a ruptured aneurysm but none was identified. In one of these there was a massive haematoma around the splenic artery and in the other five there was subarachnoid haemorrhage with additional intraventricular haemorrhage in two. Four of these cases had no autopsy and in the fifth autopsy failed to identify an aneurysm.

Ruptured aneurysms are regularly reported as a cause of maternal death. Not only is it necessary for a meticulous dissection to be performed to identify the aneurysm, often embedded in a massive haematoma, but histology is also necessary to look for features of Marfan's syndrome or of vasculitis. Histology was performed on only six of the 13 cases coming to autopsy; of the extracranial aneurysms there was histology on only two, the post-traumatic aortic aneurysm and a splenic aneurysm. In neither case was there evidence of an active vasculitis nor of Marfan's syndrome.

Comment

All cases of maternal death require a meticulous autopsy to provide not only a cause of death but also to record other pathological changes which may be present. In every case there can be no substitute for direct communication between the obstetrician and the pathologist so that the latter may be fully informed of the events leading to death. The clinical notes, with reports of all relevant investigations, should also be available.

If a hysterectomy or other surgical procedure such as salpingectomy for tubal pregnancy has been performed then preferably the excised specimen or, failing this, a report of the specimen should be submitted to the pathologist performing the autopsy. Likewise, if there is a stillborn infant this should be examined and, if appropriate, microbiological cultures taken. The placenta should be examined in all cases of maternal hypertension, antepartum or postpartum haemorrhage, and genital tract sepsis.

In cases of hypertensive disorders of pregnancy special note should be made of changes in the brain, liver and kidneys. Evidence of disseminated intravascular coagulation should be looked for and detailed histology taken of the liver, kidneys, lungs, heart, placenta and placental bed. Deaths due to antepartum or postpartum haemorrhage, in addition to detailed examination of the genital tract, require examination for amniotic fluid embolism and/or disseminated intravascular coagulation.

Where pulmonary thromboembolism is present then the likely source of the emboli should be recorded, with particular reference to whether there is thrombus in the deep veins of the calf or in the pelvic veins. Evidence of coincidental thrombosis should also be looked for in other sites, both in the venous and the arterial circulation. If there is cerebral venous thrombosis the expertise of a neuropathologist should be obtained to examine not only the brain but also the dural venous sinuses.

If amniotic fluid embolism is suspected detailed examination of the maternal pulmonary vasculature and of the parametrial and pelvic veins is required. Histological examination of several sites in the lung should be made and a minimum of five blocks from each lung is recommended. With the availability of immunohistological stains the detection of fetal squames using antibodies to cytokeratins should be a routine procedure. Examination of the buffy coat of pulmonary arterial blood is often valuable. Care must be taken in the interpretation of small quantities of lipid or mucin in the pulmonary vasculature if fetal squames are not seen.

If genital tract infection is suspected it is advisable to liaise with a microbiologist for the collection and transportation of appropriate specimens. Cultures should be taken of the fetus and placenta in addition to the genital tract and blood/splenic cultures.

Where virus infection is suspected then appropriate samples of affected tissues and blood for antibody titres should be submitted. This applies particularly to cases of myocarditis or cardiomyopathy and to cases of sudden unexplained death.

Autopsies following genital tract trauma require the obstetrician to be present from the commencement of the autopsy and both the obstetrician and the pathologist should examine the genital tract both before and after removal of the pelvic organs. If a hysterectomy has been performed then both the obstetrician and the pathologist should examine the resected specimen before it is further dissected and fixed. Opening the specimen in theatre without the pathologist present may result in failure to record important information.

Where drug therapy may be anticipated as, for example, in epilepsy, measurement of the drugs administered should be undertaken in postmortem blood samples.

However meticulous a pathologist may be in performing an autopsy, if there is inadequate communication between the obstetrician and pathologist then vital details may be lost.

The obstetrician must accept a large measure of responsibility to ensure this communication occurs.

CHAPTER 17

Recommendations

Introduction

The purpose of this chapter is to identify the principal factors contributing to maternal death, the lessons which can be learnt and clinical and administrative actions which are needed to improve care. Below we set out some of the problems and highlight the most important recommendations. General issues are considered first, followed by comments on specific clinical problems.

Many of the overall favourable trends seen in previous Reports have not been maintained. The numbers of *Direct* and *Indirect* deaths have both increased, but the number of maternities has also increased. The maternal mortality rate per 100,000 maternities, based on deaths known to the Enquiry remains unchanged compared with 1985-87 and the percentage of deaths due to maternal causes in females aged 15-44 is unchanged for the last three triennia at 0.7% (Chapter 1, Tables 1.1 and 1.2). The assessors identified evidence of substandard care in 49% cases.

These are matters of concern and there is a need for critical reappraisal of the administration and delivery of maternity care as well as the standards of clinical care.

Data collection

There have been constraints in obtaining data for this Report, some of which may be related to problems arising from NHS reorganisation. One of the main difficulties has been the initiation of Confidential Enquiries at local level. Not all Directors of Public Health Medicine see this as being within their remit and the procedure is often delegated to less experienced junior staff. The quality of clinical information has deteriorated, increasing the work of the National and Regional Assessors in making further enquiries, thus delaying the submission of forms to the Central Assessors.

It is proposed that a new United Kingdom maternal death report form be devised and that new guidelines be prepared for Directors of Public Health Medicine and for Regional Assessors to assist them in completion of Enquiries.

Death certification

Ascertainment of maternal deaths has also been more difficult because of failure to note pregnancy on death certificates, as is evident from the data in Chapter 1, and because an increasing number of deaths occur outside maternity units, in other specialist units and other Regions.

It is recommended that the death certificate form for England, Wales and Northern Ireland be modified to include a question asking whether the deceased was or had been pregnant within one year, as already pertains in Scotland and was a recommendation of the International Conference on the Classification of Diseases (10th revision) (ICD 10).

Late deaths

Although *Late* deaths are not counted for statistical purposes at present and notification was temporarily abandoned, some data was collected for the last two Reports. Reporting of *Late* deaths is at present incomplete but it is evident from the cases described in Chapter 15 that there are many such deaths in which the obstetric management had an important rôle and life was only prolonged beyond 42 days after pregnancy or delivery because of modern life support measures. There are valuable lessons to be learnt from such cases.

ICD 10 reintroduces the concept of 'Late maternal death' and it is recommended that reporting of such cases should be continued and extended to one year postpartum.

Provision of services

Purchasing health authorities have a responsibility to contract for and ensure the delivery of, and the providers have the onus to provide, high quality maternity and other specialist medical care to their population. The confidential enquiries make an important contribution to assessing standards of care and substandard care was identified in nearly half the maternal deaths.

To facilitate the conduct of the confidential enquiries Directors of Public Health Medicine need to ensure that maternal deaths are identified, enquiries initiated and data collected expeditiously and completely from all relevant sources.

Authorities should ensure, in particular, that tertiary referral services, which are likely to be regionalised, are planned for, provided and readily accessible.

Induction and updating courses for new staff

It is clear that errors often arise because of the unfamiliarity of staff with unit procedures, especially for complications which occur only infrequently, and because of a lack of a clear understanding of their own responsibilities. All staff should be instructed in the manner in which the unit operates, made familiar with the layout of the unit and be provided with up to date guidelines and protocols.

New medical and midwifery staff should have an induction course when they take up an appointment and before taking clinical responsibility. Their continuing education programme should include regular rehearsals of emergency procedures, and especially practice in cardio-pulmonary resuscitation.

Medical staffing structure

In a significant number of reported cases there is clear evidence of lack of availability of appropriate staff to deal with major problems and this has been a recurring theme of recent Reports.

There has been some increase in consultant sessions allowed for Delivery Unit supervision but the policy needs to be more widely implemented to achieve desirable levels of cover.

There is a need for continuing review of the staffing structure of obstetric units, with increased consultant involvement in acute obstetric care. Consideration should be given in each unit as to how adequate and appropriate staffing may best be achieved, taking into account local circumstances.

High dependency care and intensive therapy

Although there has been improvement in the provision of readily accessible intensive therapy facilities, there are still deficiencies in the monitoring and treatment of patients with major complications affecting fluid and electrolyte balance, particularly haemorrhage and severe pre-eclampsia and eclampsia.

There is a need to ensure that there is at least a properly equipped, staffed and supervised high dependency care area in every consultant obstetric unit. A nominated anaesthetist should be responsible for the care of patients in this area and all staff involved should receive regular training in postoperative care and resuscitation.

Domiciliary care

Adequate care in the community must be ensured for those mothers with special needs who are unable or unwilling to comply with professional advice. This involves all branches of the community care services.

For acute emergencies, such as haemorrhage or eclampsia, occurring outside hospital, appropriate expert help must be ensured. The hospital based 'Obstetric Flying Squad' is now being phased out and in many areas is defunct. Primary response to such problems is increasingly being provided by Ambulance Service Paramedics who have been appropriately trained.

In England and Wales a nationally agreed syllabus for training of paramedics in the management of obstetric emergencies is now incorporated in the NHS Training Directorate manual and is commended to Authorities.

Involvement and counselling of the mother

Mothers increasingly wish to be involved in decision making, particularly in relation to the place of delivery. For those considering having their baby away from a fully equipped consultant unit, there is a need to give a balanced appraisal of facilities which are likely to be available, those which are not, and the inevitable constraints of specialist care in such circumstances.

Many women with life threatening conditions are anxious to have children in spite of the risks involved and in the deaths reported non-compliance with professional advice was a notable feature.

There is a need to improve professional advisory and counselling skills for women with potentially life threatening conditions to ensure that both benefits and risks are clearly understood.

Hypertensive disorders of pregnancy (Chapter 2)

In this triennium there was no improvement in the maternal mortality from hypertensive disorders of pregnancy. The problems remain the same and recommendations of previous Reports have not been adequately heeded. The deficiencies are mainly organisational.

Units must have clear policies and written protocols for clinical management of hypertensive disorders of pregnancy and related complications, particularly the appropriate use of drugs and intravenous fluids, levels of responsibility and referral for specialist advice. Junior staff should be properly versed in the procedures and encouraged to refer to their consultants at an early stage.

The recommendation in previous Reports that regional centres should be identified, with staff who can give expert advice, and if necessary accept responsibility for management of cases, has so far had a disappointing response. The importance of utilising expertise in this way is again emphasised and should be addressed by purchasers and providers and management teams.

Antepartum and postpartum haemorrhage (Chapter 3)

The number of deaths from haemorrhage increased in this triennium and substandard care was a major feature. The need for a team approach to the management of severe haemorrhage is apparently not adequately recognised.

Those units which do not have a written protocol for the management of massive haemorrhage are recommended to consider the Revised Guidelines provided as an annexe to Chapter 3 of this Report.

The majority of consultant units now have a blood bank and intensive therapy facilities on site, and have protocols for the management of massive haemorrhage. Although management guidelines were given in the previous Report, 18% units still lack a written protocol.

High priority should be given to remedying any remaining deficiencies in service provision, particularly the availability of blood in smaller units. Attention should be given to the organisation of staff and contingency plans to cope with sudden unexpected haemorrhage.

Thrombosis and thromboembolism (Chapter 4)

The number of deaths from thromboembolism after vaginal delivery has fallen but deaths in the antenatal period and after Caesarean section continue to cause concern.

There have been no appropriate randomised controlled trials in relation to prevention of thrombo-embolic complications. The dangers of anticoagulant therapy may have been exaggerated and their rôle in prophylaxis and in cases where the diagnosis is in doubt, together with other prophylactic measures, should be reconsidered.

Awareness of the possible diagnosis of thromboembolic disorders could be improved and more use should be made of the better diagnostic tests which are now available. There is a clear need for further research in this area, particularly in relation to prophylaxis.

Early pregnancy deaths (Chapter 6)

There continue to be problems in the management of early pregnancy complications, resulting both from lack of senior supervision and reluctance of junior staff, both obstetric and anaesthetic, to request assistance. Follow up is deficient in some cases, including review of pathology findings.

The clinical history and findings in cases of ectopic pregnancy are often equivocal and careful assessment and follow up in such cases is mandatory. The recommendations made in the previous Report are re-emphasised and they are reproduced in Chapter 6.

Genital tract sepsis (Chapter 7)

When sepsis associated with deaths in early pregnancy is included there was an increase in the number of deaths due to sepsis in this triennium.

Microbiological investigation was often incomplete and initiated too late. Full details of antibiotic therapy were rarely available to the assessors but in several cases it was evident that therapy was not sufficiently aggressive.

There is no general agreement on the use of routine prophylactic antibiotics at the time of Caesarean section, although Enkin et al (1989) conclude that '...the evidence we have reviewed justifies far wider adoption of antibiotic prophylaxis than currently exists.'

The importance of seeking advice from a microbiologist at an early stage in the management of sepsis is again emphasised.

Deaths associated with anaesthesia and postoperative care (Chapter 9)

The number of deaths directly due to complications of anaesthesia was the lowest ever recorded. It is believed that this is largely due to the implementation of recommendations made in previous Reports.

Anaesthesia and deficiencies in postoperative care contributed to a number of other deaths. In particular 44 deaths were due to the Adult Respiratory Distress Syndrome or associated complications. Significant predisposing factors were haemorrhage or severe hypotension, aspiration of gastric contents, chest infection, sepsis and hypertensive disorders of pregnancy.

[Enkin M *et al*, in *'Effective Care in Pregnancy and Childbirth'* ed. Chalmers I, Enkin M and Keirse MJMC. Ch 73, p.1265 Oxford: Oxford University Press, 1989.]

H^2 receptor blocking drugs should be administered to all patients who are likely to require anaesthesia and to patients with severe pre-eclampsia. A non-particulate antacid should also be given before induction of general anaesthesia. In patients in whom delayed gastric emptying is suspected, preoperative emptying of the stomach should be considered. Also the stomach should be routinely emptied before the patient recovers from the anaesthetic to minimise the risks of postoperative aspiration.

Attention must be given to the improvement of perioperative care. All patients should be monitored by pulse oximetry during operation and in the immediate postoperative period, and such monitoring should be continued if there is a possibility of a deterioration in the patient's condition. When severe haemorrhage is observed or suspected wide bore IV cannulae and a CVP line should be inserted and the assistance of senior obstetric, anaesthetic and blood transfusion staff requested immediately.

Although the majority of obstetric units are now well supervised by consultant anaesthetists, there are still a number of units in which there is inadequate consultant supervision and training of junior staff.

Adequate consultant supervision is difficult to achieve when anaesthetic departments are small or in obstetric units isolated from the main hospital. Every effort should be made to transfer isolated consultant units to major hospital sites.

Other Direct deaths (Chapter 10)

The number of other *Direct* deaths has fallen but in more than half the cases the cause of death was not adequately explained. If this unsatisfactory state of affairs is to be rectified complete and accurate clinical and autopsy records must be available for study in every case (See also Chapter 16).

Medical and surgical disorders (Chapters 11 & 12)

Pregnancies associated with medical and surgical disorders continue to be a major problem in obstetric practice and in a high proportion of cases there is substandard care. There is often failure to recognise a disorder or to appreciate its significance in relation to pregnancy.

There is evidence of failure of diagnosis and of inappropriate assessment of the severity of the disorder in several cases. Proper clinical examination is essential and specialist opinion should be obtained if there is any element of doubt. Diagnoses based on assessments made several years previously and without the benefit of modern techniques should not be readily accepted and all such cases should be reappraised.

There is a need for more effective pre-pregnancy counselling of women with medical and surgical problems and, for those who elect to become pregnant, expert supervision and combined care with a specialist in the particular condition is essential.

During and immediately after delivery is a particularly hazardous period, particularly for women with cardiac disease, and specialist help and facilities must be readily available at this time.

In all pregnant women with medical or surgical disorders consideration should be given to the best place for antenatal care and for delivery, ensuring proximity to intensive therapy and other specialist services relevant to the particular case. As an emergency situation may arise at any time there should be adequate contingency plans which are clearly understood by staff on duty.

Caesarean section (Chapter 13)

The number of deaths associated with Caesarean section increased but the number of unplanned emergency operations decreased and substandard care was less common.

The main features of substandard care remain the same: inappropriate delegation, inadequate consultation and inadequate support facilities. In particular deaths from haemorrhage were often associated with high risk cases delivered by junior medical staff.

Attention is again drawn to the poor fetal outcome following postmortem Caesarean section, with no surviving babies in the eight cases reported. All staff who might be involved with such problems need to have clear guidelines on appropriate management of sudden death in pregnancy.

Pathology

Autopsies were performed in 81% cases but deficiencies in the quality of the examinations, particularly in relation to histology, microbiology and toxicology, persist. This is especially so in cases under the jurisdiction of the Coroner/Fiscal which now account for about 90% all maternal autopsies.

The essential requirements for a maternal autopsy are set out in Chapter 16 and should be followed.

The educational value of the autopsy should not be overlooked and clinicians should always be present to discuss the findings with the pathologist.

CHAPTER 18

Maternal Mortality in Europe

Introduction

Crude maternal death rates are available for all countries in Europe and comparisons are often based on such data. However there is little information readily available on the denominators, definitions, registration and verification procedures on which such data is based. This review attempts to collate such information as could be obtained in order to encourage more meaningful comparisons in the future.

Several possible European and international sources were approached as potential repositories of the appropriate information concerning denominators and criteria used but no single source could provide such information. It was therefore decided to approach likely organisations in individual countries and a questionnaire (Appended) was sent to the National Administrators of the member countries of the European College of Obstetrics and Gynaecology (ECOG), with the approval and support of the Council of the College, and to the Secretaries of all the national societies of Obstetrics and Gynaecology. We are grateful for the support of ECOG and for the responses and data we have received from our European colleagues.

World Health Organisation Data

The International Classification of Diseases 9th Revision (ICD 9) definition of maternal death is:

> "...death of a woman while pregnant or within 42 days of pregnancy, irrespective of the duration and the site of the pregnancy, from any cause related to or aggravated by the pregnancy or its management but not from accidental or incidental causes.
>
> Maternal deaths should be divided into two groups:
>
> 1) Direct obstetric deaths: Those resulting from obstetric complications of the pregnant state (pregnancy, labour and the puerperium), from interventions, omissions, incorrect treatment, or from a chain of events resulting from any of the above.
>
> 2) Indirect obstetric deaths: Those resulting from previous existing disease that developed during pregnancy and which was not due to direct causes, but which was aggravated by physiologic effects of pregnancy."

The WHO collects statistics in certain broad categories based on ICD 9 codings and these are available from Eurostat (Health for All 2000, WHO 1991). The latest available data is summarised in Table 18.1. Maternal mortality rates for Western Europe are around 10/100,000 live births. Generally the rates in Scandinavian countries have been about half this figure and in Mediterranean countries rates have been higher. The highest rates have been in Eastern Europe, with the highest recorded rate being in Romania.

The European Survey

The purpose of this survey was to endeavour to ascertain the degree of uniformity in data collection and analysis in Europe. Questionnaires were sent to the National representatives of all the member countries of the European College of Obstetricians and Gynaecologists and to the secretaries of National Societies. Data was sought from 20 countries and replies were received from 17.

Definitions

All but one of the respondents stated that ICD 9 was used for definitions and classification; one country (Switzerland) still used ICD 8. However there were significant deviations in detail. The commonest was the inclusion of *Fortuitous* deaths in the statistical data in seven countries (Finland, Hungary, Iceland, Irish Republic, Malta, Norway [some], Romania). *Late deaths* were included in five countries (Iceland, Irish Republic, Netherlands, Norway[some], Switzerland). *Deaths from abortion and ectopic gestation* were excluded in one country (Irish Republic) and deaths in which the fetus was less than 30cm long in one country (Switzerland).

Identification of maternal deaths

All countries had a national data collection agency and in some countries there were one or more regional agencies which tended to produce more complete and reliable data. Various secondary checks were used in different countries, including statutory notification separate from the general death notification system, culling of hospital reports, personal local knowledge resulting from enquiry studies and verification of death certificates for all deaths in women of child bearing age.

In only four countries (Denmark, Germany, Irish Republic, Scotland) does the death certificate contain a specific question on pregnancy.

To facilitate identification of maternal deaths the new ICD 10 introduces a new category of *pregnancy related death*, defined as:

> *"the death of a woman while pregnant or within 42 days of termination of pregnancy, irrespective of the cause of death"* and is intended *"for use where the cause of death cannot be identified precisely."*

National Enquiries

Five countries (Hungary, Irish Republic, Netherlands, Romania, United Kingdom,) carried out enquiries into individual deaths but in four countries there were enquiries centred on some or all regions (Belgium, France, Germany, Norway). The nature of the enquiries ranged from a detailed confidential analysis, as in the United Kingdom, to a quasi-judicial investigation with risk of criminal proceedings, as in Romania. The results of the Enquiries were not necessarily published.

Autopsies

Verification of cause of death by autopsy varied but was sometimes a statutory obligation. In the majority of countries autopsies were performed in over 75% cases but in three countries (France, Irish Republic, Spain) the rate was less than 50%. The autopsy was reputedly carried out by a pathologist with special experience in maternal pathology in seven countries (Finland, Germany, Hungary, Iceland, Romania, Spain, Switzerland) but in three of these the number of maternal deaths averaged five or less per annum (Finland, Iceland, Switzerland).

Evidence of under-reporting

It is generally recognised that under-reporting of maternal deaths is common, even in countries with sophisticated registration systems and, for example, in Table 18.1 zero returns, which are particularly common in the category "Other *Indirect* obstetric deaths", may be due to small numbers or to failure to collect the data. There may be a number of factors contributing to under-recording. Zahr and Royston (1991) identified certain general contributory influences such as social, religious, emotional and practical factors, including desire to avoid blame. More specific factors concerned with registration include:

>i. Maternal deaths may not be identified because of coding errors and ambiguities. For example there is ambiguity in coding deaths from certain causes, such as cerebral haemorrhage which may be coded as 'Diseases of the circulatory system' (430-434) or as a complication of pregnancy (648.6 or 674), (See data of Bouvier-Colle et al, below).

>ii. Poor denominator data.

>iii. The use of different denominators, such as the number of women of reproductive age or the number of live births, even though with the latter the numerator is likely to include women having stillbirths or dying from early pregnancy complications.

>iv. The exclusion of conditions which are included in the ICD 9 definition, such as early pregnancy deaths and *Indirect* deaths

Table 18.1 *Maternal deaths in Europe* Rates per 100,000 livebirths

COUNTRY	YEAR	All causes 630: 676	Abortion 630: 639	Haemorrhage 640 641 666	'Toxaemia' 642.4: 642.9 643	Puerperium 670: 676	Other Direct Obstetric 646.6 660	Other Indirect Obstetric 647 648 650
Austria*	89	7.89	1.13	2.25	2.25	1.13	1.13	0
Belgium	86	3.42°	0.85	0	0.85	0.85	0.85	0
Bulgaria	89	18.70	5.34	6.23	1.78	2.67	2.67	0
Czechoslovakia	89	9.59	1.92	1.44	0.48	2.88	2.40	0.48
DDR	89	11.56	0	1.01	2.64	4.02	0	0
Denmark*	88	3.40°	0	0	3.40	0	0	0
FDR	89	5.28	0.44	0.44	1.17	2.05	0.73	0.44
Finland*	88	11.06°	3.16	3.16	0	3.16	0	1.58
France	88	9.34	0.39	1.17	1.43	1.94	4.02	0.39
Greece	88	5.58°	0.93	0	2.79	0.93	0.93	0
Hungary	89	15.41	2.43	0.81	0.81	3.24	7.30	0.81
Iceland**	89	0°						
Irish Republic*	88	1.83°	0	0	0	1.83	0	0
Israel*	87	3.03	0	0	0	2.02	1.01	0
Italy	88	7.63	1.04	2.43	1.39	0.69	1.91	0.17
Luxembourg**	89	0°	0	0	0	0	0	0
Malta**	89	0°	0	0	0	0	0	0
Monaco**	87	0°	0	0	0	0	0	0
Netherlands	88	9.64	1.07	1.07	3.75	1.61	1.61	0.54

Table 18.1 *Maternal deaths in Europe (cont)*

COUNTRY	YEAR	All causes 630: 676	Abortion 630: 639	Haemorrhage 640 641 666	'Toxaemia' 642.4: 642.9 643	Puerperium 670: 676	Other Direct Obstetric 646.6 660	Other Indirect Obstetric 647 648 650
Norway*	88	3.48°	0	1.74	1.74	0	0	0
Poland	89	10.67	2.31	1.42	1.24	3.73	0.18	0.36
Portugal	89	10.12	4.22	1.69	0.84	0.84	2.53	0
Romania	84	148.83	128.01	4.85	3.14	8.55	4.28	0
Spain	86	5.47	0.68	0.91	0.68	2.05	1.14	0
Sweden	87	4.78°	0	0	0.96	1.91	1.91	0
Switzerland	89	3.70°	0	0	2.46	1.23	0	0
Turkey	90	130	–	–	–	–	–	–
USSR	89	43.83	10.43	6.99	5.02	–	–	–
United Kingdom	89	7.72	0.77	0.90	1.54	1.67	1.54	1.29
Italy	88	7.63	1.04	2.43	1.39	0.69	1.91	0.17
Yugoslavia	88	16.28	3.93	2.25	3.15	1.68	0	0
EUROPE		16.64	8.41	1.69	1.50	2.34	1.73	0.36

* Less than 100,000 live births per annum

** Less than 50,000 live births per annum.

o Five or less reported maternal deaths per annum.

DATA FROM: *Health for All 2000.* WHO, Geneva (1991)
Maternal Health: A Global Factbook. WHO, Geneva (1991)

(although in some countries the numbers may be inflated by the inclusion of *Fortuitous* and *Late* deaths).

v. Lack of verification and back up systems for identifying cases and confirmation of cause of death, especially when death does not occur in an obstetric unit.

vi. Death due to direct causes may be delayed beyond 42 days because of the use of modern life support measures.

Data derived from official statistics has been shown to be unreliable in many studies in the United States of America and in certain European countries. Bouvier-Colle et al (1991) reviewed a number of surveys in Europe and the USA which showed underestimation of maternal deaths ranging from 17% to 62.8%.

In the United Kingdom the returns from the Registrar General for the years 1988-90 identified 173 maternal deaths due to 'a complication of pregnancy, childbirth or the puerperium' whereas the Confidential Enquiry identified 238 *Direct* and *Indirect* deaths, 38% more than the official statistics. (See Chapter 1).

In France Bouvier-Colle et al (1991) carried out a retrospective survey of 3045 deaths of women aged 15-44 years. Sixty eight deaths were in pregnant or puerperal women and of these 54 had obstetric causes. In only 41 deaths had complications of pregnancy or the puerperium been recorded on the death certificate and only 24 had been allocated to ICD 9 maternal mortality codes. This suggests an under-reporting of 56% in the official statistics.

In Germany no records have been kept since reunification in 1989 but in Bavaria there is an ongoing detailed analysis based on the UK Confidential Enquiries format, with publication planned for 1993. All deaths of women of child bearing age are checked and it is believed that the coverage is virtually complete.

Conclusion

This review, by identifying current problems, can be regarded as a first step towards obtaining some valid European comparisons on Maternal Mortality based on uniformity of data collection, verification and analysis. It highlights discrepancies in classification although all countries purported to base their analysis on ICD 9 definitions and codings.

Many of the difficulties identified would be alleviated by incorporating in death certificates an annotated box specifically asking (for female deaths) whether the woman was pregnant or had been within the six weeks prior to death, as is the current practice in Scotland.

To facilitate identification of maternal deaths the new ICD 10 introduces a new category of *pregnancy related death*, defined as:

> *"the death of a woman while pregnant or within 42 days of termination of pregnancy, irrespective of the cause of death" and is intended "for use where the cause of death cannot be identified precisely."*

In order to include deaths in which life has been prolonged by life sustaining procedures ICD 10 also reintroduces the category of *Late* maternal death, defined as:

> *"the death of a woman from direct and indirect obstetric causes more than 42 days but less than one year after termination of pregnancy"*

Data currently available should be interpreted with extreme caution, especially when attempting international comparisons and a more effective mechanism for ensuring uniformity of data should be established within the European Community.

References

Bouvier-Colle M-H, Varnoux N, Costes P, Hatton F: Reasons for the underreporting of Maternal Mortality in France, as indicated by a survey of all deaths among women of childbearing age. *International Journal of Epidemiology* 1991; **20:** 717–721

WHO. *Health for All 2000* Geneva: WHO, 1991.

WHO. *International Classification of Diseases 9th Revision*. Geneva: WHO, 1977.

Abou Zar C., Royston E: *Maternal Mortality — a Global Factbook*. Geneva: WHO, 1991.

APPENDIX

Questionnaire sent to all National Administrators of ECOG and Secretaries of National Societies

Maternal Mortality Surveillance — a European Comparison

COUNTRY

RESPONDENT

Maternal mortality rate for latest available 3 years   19...

19...

19...

Do you have any data on the main causes of maternal death?

Definitions

Classification used   ICD9 / Other
  (If other please detail)

Are the following included?
  Abortion (spontaneous or therapeutic)   Yes/No
  Other gestational age criteria   Yes/No
  If 'Yes' — specify....................................

  Ectopic gestation   Yes/No
  Indirect deaths (i.e. due to pre-existing
  disease but aggravated by pregnancy)   Yes/No
  Fortuitous deaths (i.e. coincidental,
    e.g. road accident)   Yes/No
  Dying undelivered   Yes/No
  Death within 42 days post partum   Yes/No
  Death after 42 days post partum   Yes/No
  If 'No' - specify.....................................

Autopsy

In approximately what proportion of deaths is a postmortem
examination performed? >75%

50-75%

<50%

Does the pathologist usually have special experience in
maternal autopsies? Yes/No

Data collection

Does the national death certificate have a separate box to
indicate pregnancy? Yes/No

What is your national agency for data collection?....................

What verification mechanisms do you have?.........................

What additional safeguards do you have to ensure ascertainment is as
complete as possible? (e.g. are death certificates which give cause of
death as pulmonary embolism questioned?; Are there any safeguards
to ensure notification of maternal deaths which occur outside a maternity unit?)

Do you have a national enquiry into maternal deaths? Yes/No
If so please give brief details of organisation

Any other observations?

Thank you for your help. We will send you a copy of the collated data
in due course.

Acknowledgements

This Report has been made possible by the help and work of the District Directors of Public Health in England and Chief Administrative Medical Officers in Wales, Scotland and Northern Ireland who initiated case reports and collected the information, and the consultant obstetricians, anaesthetists and pathologists, general practitioners and midwives who have supplied the detailed case records and autopsy reports.

Considerable assistance has also been given by procurators fiscal who have supplied copies of reports of autopsies, and by coroners who have supplied autopsy reports and sometimes inquest proceedings to the assessors.

The staff of the Medical Statistics Division of the Office of Population Censuses and Surveys in England have worked with the information and Statistics Division of the Common Services Agency in Scotland [and departmental statisticians in Wales and Northern Ireland] to prepare the Introduction to the Report, process the statistical data and prepare the Tables and Figures.

The Editorial Board would like to express their thanks to all these people and also in particular to the consultant obstetricians, anaesthetists and pathologists listed below who have acted as regional assessors in England and assessors in Scotland and helped in the preparation of this Report.

The assessors for Wales and Northern Ireland are members of the Editorial Board and are listed on page iv.

I. ENGLISH REGIONAL ASSESSORS IN OBSTETRICS

Northern Region	Professor W Dunlop FRCS FRCOG
Yorkshire Region	Mr A G Gordon FRCS FRCOG
Trent Region	Professor J MacVicar MD FRCS FRCOG
East Anglian Region	Mr J A Carron Brown FRCS FRCOG
	Mr P J Milton MA MD FRCOG, from Oct 1992
North West Thames Region	Mr A C Fraser FRCOG
North East Thames Region	Professor H A Brant MD FRCS(Ed) FRCP(Ed) FRCOG
	Mr M Setchell FRCS FRCOG, from Oct 1992
South East Thames Region	Mr E D Morris MD FRCS FRCOG

South West Thames Region	Professor G V P Chamberlain MD FRCS FRCOG
Oxford Region	Mr G Mitford Barberton FRCOG
	Mr M Gillmer MD FRCOG, from Oct 1990
South Western Region	Professor G M Stirrat MA MD FRCOG
West Midlands Region:	Mr H Oliphant Nicholson FRCS FRCOG
North Western Region	Mr P Donnai MA MB BChir FRCOG
Mersey Region	Mrs S H Towers MD FRCOG
Wessex Region	Professor John Dennis FRCS FRCOG (declared Dec 1989)
	Mr C P Jardine Brown FRCS FRCOG, from April 1990

II. ENGLISH REGIONAL ANAESTHETIC ASSESSORS

Northern Region	Dr M R Bryson MB BS FFARCS
Yorkshire Region	Dr F Richard Ellis PhD MB ChB FFARCS
Trent Region	Dr A Caunt MB ChB FFARCS
East Anglian Region	Dr B R Wilkey BM BCh FFARCS
North West Thames Region	Dr M Morgan MB BS FFARCS
North East Thames Region	Dr Hilary Howells MB ChB FFARCS
	Dr Miriam Frank FFARCS, from Nov 1990
South East Thames Region	Dr P B Hewitt MB BS FFARCS
South West Thames Region	Dr H F Seeley MSc MA MB BS FFARCS
Oxford Region	Dr Edmonds Seal MB BS FFARCS
South Western Region	Dr T A Thomas MB ChB FFARCS
West Midlands Region	Dr A M Veness MB ChB FFARCS
North Western Region	Dr J M Anderton MB ChB FFARCS
Mersey Region	Dr T H L Bryson MB ChB FFARCS
Wessex Region	Professor John Norman PhD FFARCS

III. ENGLISH REGIONAL ASSESSORS IN PATHOLOGY

Northern Region	Dr E W Walton MD FRCPath
	Dr A R Morley MD FRCPath
Yorkshire Region	Dr I N Reid MB ChB FRCPath
Trent Region	Dr A Shirley Hill MA FRCP FRCOG FRCPath
East Anglian Region	Dr Phillip F Roberts MB BS MRCP FRCPath
North West Thames Region	Dr I A Lampert MB ChB DCP FRCPath
North East Thames Region	Dr R G M Letcher MB BS FRCPath
	Dr J Crow BSc MB BS FRCPath, from Nov 1990
South East Thames Region	Dr M Driver MB BS FRCPath
	Dr Nigel Kirkham MB ChB MRCPath, from Nov 1990
South West Thames Region	Dr N Hall MB BS MRCPath
Oxford Region	Dr W Gray MB BS FRCPath
South Western Region	Professor P P Anthony MB BS FRCPath

West Midlands Region	Dr D I Rushton MB ChB FRCPath
North Western Region	Professor H Fox MD FRCPath
Mersey Region	Dr I W McDicken MD FRCPath
Wessex Region	Dr G H Millward-Sadler BSc MB ChB FRCPath

IV. SCOTTISH ASSESSORS TO THE CEMD NOT SERVING ON THE UK CEMD EDITORIAL BOARD

Dr M H Hall MD MBChB FRCOG)
Dr N B Patel MBChB FRCOG)
Dr J B Scrimgeour MBChB FRCS FRCOG) Obstetric
Dr K S Stewart MD MBChB FRCS FRCOG)
Dr H P McEwan MD MBChB FRCS FRCOG)
Dr J Thorburn MBChB FFARCS DObstRCOG Anaesthetic

Printed in the United Kingdom for HMSO.
Dd.0297617, 12/93, C80, 3396/4, 5673, 267988.